THE VIEW
FROM THE VUE

THE VIEW FROM THE VUE

Larry Karp

Originally published by Jonathan David Publishers

Copyright © 1977, 2000 by Larry Karp

ISBN: 978-1-5040-3613-9

Distributed in 2016 by Open Road Distribution
180 Maiden Lane
New York, NY 10038
www.openroadmedia.com

FOR MYRA

Preface

One day in the autumn of 1958, I went for an interview to New York University School of Medicine. N.Y.U.'s major affiliated teaching facility was (and still is) Bellevue Hospital. During the course of my interview, the Dean asked me why I wanted to go to medical school. I told him:

> I want to be a doctor because then I'll have an acceptable excuse to talk and listen to unusual people for the rest of my life. I want to come to Bellevue because I think that's where they have more unusual people than anywhere else in the world.

The Dean cleared his throat, and I jumped out of my chair. But then I saw the corners of his mouth flickering upward, and I heard him say:

> You know, we get pretty weary of hearing one applicant after the other say he wants to become a doctor so that he can help suffering humanity. You are either terribly honest or terribly inventive. Either way, you're so far out I feel you can't help but succeed.

I thanked the Dean and went home. My letter of acceptance arrived three days later.

So, I went to Bellevue. During the next six years, as medical student, intern, and resident physician, I watched in gratified amazement as great giant hordes of peculiar individuals acted out their scenes before me. I had been right: there seemed to be something in those dingy wards and hallways that brought out the exceptional in the inhabitants, whether they were patients, relatives, or hospital employees.

When the new Bellevue Hospital, twelve years in the building, finally opened a few years ago, alumni throughout America sighed in relief and offered the opinion that life at The Vue would henceforth be very different. But I knew better. It didn't matter that the physical structure was new, because the hospital would continue to be inhabited by the very same cast of characters who had always caused Bellevue to be a singularity, and who always will.

This is a book about the singular people of Bellevue Hospital.

LAURENCE E. KARP

Table of Contents

Introduction

An Overview
of The Vue

We called it THE VUE, and without a doubt that was the most complimentary nickname Bellevue Hospital ever had. More than once I heard someone call the place Bedlam Hospital, after the infamous London madhouse. Other sobriquets were even more derogatory. In the process of interviewing an internship candidate, one of the residents referred to his place of employment as Satan's Little Acre. And one day, as I got up to debark from a bus pulling to a stop in front of Bellevue, the driver sang out, "Foist Av'noo'n Twenty-six Street. Noo Yawk City Slaughterhouse."

There existed many reasons for the plethora of nasty names. Throughout its very long history Bellevue has traditionally dispensed free medical care to the needy, and people generally feel that anything free is worth no more than the price. Bellevue has long been associated with medical schools; hence it became known as the place where innocent patients were butchered by students while learning their trade. Then too, The Vue possessed a well-earned reputation as an outstanding research center which, unfortunately, gave rise to the belief that if you were lucky enough to escape the blunders of its medical students, some nut in a long white coat would turn you into a guinea pig. Nor did certain of Bellevue's component parts help its image; for any huge general hospital which also happens to contain within its walls both a major psychiatric institution and the city morgue is more likely to inspire trepidation than adulation in the minds of the local populace.

Perhaps as much as anything, Bellevue's very appearance was responsible for its lack of charisma. Many of today's medical centers, especially those seen on television, are soaring glass-and-concrete architectural triumphs, designed to lead people to imagine that the gods of healing truly do reside there. In contrast, Bellevue appeared to have been constructed by a man whose mother had been frightened by a Picasso drawing of a toad.

Set down on a rectangular plot bordered by the East River Drive, First Avenue, Twenty-sixth Street, and Thirtieth Street, The Vue was a dreadful melange of squat buildings of dark red and dirty yellow brick. The various edifices were put up between 1904 and 1940, each part a seeming afterthought, connected to the others by endless mazes of hallways and subterranean tunnels. The entire complex was surrounded by a black iron fence. An uninformed visitor to New York City, on seeing the hospital, would most likely have assumed it to be a prison built especially for the detention of the most despicable and miserable sorts of criminals.

If such a visitor were sufficiently courageous to set appearances aside and walk into the hospital, he would have been even more dismayed. Entering through the main door, he'd have found himself in a large lobby, consisting of a wide walkway running past a line of information cages, whose bars reinforced the general prison-like appearance of the institution. On the other side of the walkway, and occupying most of the lobby area, he'd have seen rows of brown wooden benches. Most of the seats would have been occupied by as colorful a representation of the lower socioeconomic classes as one could possibly find anywhere on earth.

Bowery bums would have been scattered here and there, mostly sitting hunched forward, staring at the floor. Perhaps one, his head wrapped in bandages and gauze, would have been lying on his side, his knees drawn up to his chest and his mouth hanging slackly open. Nearby, but at a discreet distance, an old woman with a shawl over her stringy gray hair might have been sitting with a shopping bag between her feet, her eyes darting back and forth as though on guard against an imminent assault. Three benches away, there could have been a junkie, nodding off to sleep. Around them all, large numbers of ragged little children of all sizes and colors would have been charging back and forth, playing tag and chasing each other between the benches. Occasionally, the old woman would have become irritated and shooed some of them off. They'd have laughed at her and continued their games. The visitor would have wrinkled his nose against the stench of unwashed bodies and exhaled alcohol.

Proceeding past the lobby and through the labyrinthine halls, the visitor to New York would have come upon one or another of the patient areas. Private rooms were a rarity at The Vue, the few that existed usually being reserved for sick doctors or nurses who chose to be treated on their home grounds. Open wards were the rule; they contained anywhere from twenty to forty beds in two or three long rows stretching the length of the room. Curtains could be pulled around the beds at the sides of the ward, but privacy was impossible to the inhabitants of the center row.

Everything in the place was in disrepair. Cobwebs and dirt hung in the corners between the high walls and the ceilings. No wall was without its region of peeling paint or plaster. The hands on the flyspecked clocks stood motionless, except for the occasional pair that zoomed through hours in seconds, giving off a buzzing noise as they did. Lighting was dim throughout, and dark shadows that moved slowly across the walls, floors, and ceilings produced an atmosphere of depression which continually affected the mood and behavior of the inhabitants.

Right from its beginning, Bellevue was Bellevue. The institution dates its origins, spiritually, if not physically, to 1736 when a six-bed infirmary was set up in the New York Publick Workhouse and House of Correction, located in the region of the present-day entrance to the Brooklyn Bridge. There, the medical and surgical needs of the inmate prisoners and indigents were attended to.

As early as 1811, New York was beginning to show signs of growing pains, so the city purchased a large farm on what was then uptown land, near the East River. A part of this region was known as Belle Vue (which it may well have been at the time), and the public hospital facility constructed on the site took its name from the location. Like the city it served, it grew like Topsy.

By 1877, one hundred years ago, The Vue had twelve hundred beds, an emergency room, ambulance services, and outpatient facilities. (These latter three attributes were all Bellevue innovations.) It even had its own medical school: after a decade during which lectures and surgical demonstrations were presented on a loosely organized basis, the Bellevue Hospital Medical College was founded in 1861. This marked the formal beginning of The Vue as a teaching institution, a *modus operandi* which has persisted to the present day. But not via the same vehicle. Little more than thirty years after it had begun operations, the physical plant of the Bellevue Medical School was destroyed by fire. The faculty then accepted the offer of the nearby New York University Medical College to share its facilities and, in 1898, the Bellevue people decided to merge with their benefactors rather than rebuild. Thus began the association between N.Y.U. and The Vue, which has continued without interruption for the past seventy-nine years.

During this interval, Bellevue has been the focal point of many historic medical crises and catastrophes. During the early years of the twentieth century, there were several spectacular fires in lower Manhattan. When the steamer *General Slocum* burned in the East River in 1904, more than a thousand of its passengers were killed and several hundred were injured. The majority of these survivors were brought to The Vue by horse-drawn ambulances. The same equine-powered conveyances also brought in the victims of the 1911 Triangle Shirtwaist Company fire and the 1912 Equitable Life Assurance Building conflagration.

The year 1918 marked the great influenza epidemic, and the lion's share of the seriously ill New Yorkers received their inpatient care at The Vue. Since there was no effective treatment for the condition, mortality rates were astronomical: on one particular day that fall, sixty-two Bellevue inmates lost their battle with the flu bug. Included among the grim statistics were several members of the hospital's nursing and physician staffs.

In the spring of 1947, New York City had a serious smallpox scare. The disease was brought in by a traveler from Mexico who, on his way to Maine, got as far as Gotham before collapsing. Guess where he went for help at that point. Before the problem was declared solved, two months had passed, twelve people had come down with smallpox (two of whom died), six million citizens had been vaccinated, and the city had spent more than $800,000 to prevent the generalized epidemic which otherwise would certainly have occurred.

Around the turn of the century, it became apparent that the physical facilities were grossly inadequate for the medical load, and what was left of the grass and trees from old Belle Vue began to disappear under tons of brick and mortar. New buildings were erected in 1904, 1908, 1911, 1916, and 1917. In 1926, Mayor Jimmy Walker referred to the psychiatric facilities as "a state of affairs in which I wouldn't ask my dog to be kept." Four years later, Beau James presided at the ground-breaking ceremonies for the new psychiatry pavilion, which was opened in 1935. Lastly, the administration building, at the front and near the middle of the complex, was completed in 1940. With that, almost every inch of space was occupied, with the exception of a parking lot in the back.

But Manhattan continued to outgrow The Vue, and by the early 1960's, New York City's Municipal and Hospital administrations reached the decision that the conglomeration of now old buildings could no longer be tolerated, and that an entire new Bellevue must be built. That was the end of the parking lot. Having the unmistakable evidence of wisdom of brick-and-mortar neighbors on all sides that proved the folly of wasting air space in twentieth-century New York City, the administrators and the architects resolved that Nova Bellevue would scrape the sky like all modern structures, and thereby require a minimum of ground space. A deep hole was sunk into the turf where Pontiacs and Volkswagens had once pranced, and there it remained for several years, periodically filling up with water, awaiting the resolution of multiplex municipal squabbles that delayed construction progress. But finally, in 1966, construction was resumed, and after seven more years had passed the new building was dedicated. All things take time. Especially at Bellevue.

My tenure at The Vue essentially spanned the hole-in-the-ground years. I arrived as a first-year medical student in the fall of 1959, and left (at the insistence of my tall, bewhiskered uncle) after a year of residency, in 1965. Since first- and second-year medical students spent little time on the wards, my intense and intimate association with the place actually covered a four-year period, consisting of most of the early 1960's, a time of great social upheaval and turmoil in American society.

As the primary municipal hospital in Manhattan, The Vue drew patients from the entire borough, although the great majority of the clientele came from lower Manhattan. This region included the Bowery and its numerous derelicts who were accustomed to patronizing The Vue to obtain medical repair of their worn-out parts (usually lungs or livers).

Many Bellevue patients came from the Lower East Side of Manhattan. The Lower East Siders consisted primarily of two groups of people. First, there were the elderly Jews, the holdovers from the massive wave of Middle and Eastern European immigrants who had come to America earlier in the twentieth century, and who had turned large areas of the Lower East Side into mini-ghettos. Their children moved on to New Jersey or Long Island, but the old people remained where they had grown up and raised their families. Each year there were fewer of them, but their numbers were still considerable. The other major Lower East Side group was made up of more recent immigrants, the Puerto Ricans. Often, whole families resettled en masse in New York, and infirm Puerto Ricans kept all the Bellevue wards busy, from pediatrics to geriatrics.

As in its earliest days, Bellevue generally catered to the less-solvent strata of society, but such was not invariably the case. Sometimes, The Vue would play host to a middle-class or even an affluent patient. This was especially likely to happen in case of emergencies, such as when a neighborhood businessman suffered a heart attack while at work, or when a suburban housewife, in the city for a day of shopping, misjudged the determination of a cab driver while crossing the street, and was brought in with tread marks on her person. And additionally, since one's social or financial status is never a factor when one runs amuck, some fairly "fancy" people were taken to Bellevue Psychiatric Hospital for observation.

At the other end of the social spectrum, The Vue never forgot its Publick Workhouse and House of Correction origins, and a portion of the second floor was set aside as a prison ward, complete with barred doors and windows, with police on duty in addition to the usual ward attendants. Here prisoners were brought from the various New York jails whose medical or surgical problems could not be handled by the jail infirmaries.

All members of the Bellevue medical staff were affiliated with a medical school, thereby making The Vue a teaching hospital. During the early 1960's, three schools provided The Vue with its students and staff. Bellevue was the primary teaching facility for New York University, but Columbia and Cornell both maintained very active secondary affiliations. (Their primary associations were with Presbyterian and New York Hospital, respectively.) Today only N.Y.U. is represented at The Vue. By reducing the number of medical indigents in the city, health insurance has lowered Bellevue's patient population to the point where it can no longer support more than one medical school.

The medical personnel at Bellevue were organized along rigid hierarchical lines. Low men on the totem pole were the freshman and sophomore students. During their first two years of training, most of their time was spent in classrooms, learning the principles of basic medical science. On occasion, groups of them were brought together with experienced doctors on the Bellevue wards, to be taught the skills of physical diagnosis. This first experience in the bowels of the Behemoth of First Avenue was usually more or less unnerving to the initiates, which was made apparent by their pale faces and nervously darting eyes.

By the third year of medical school, students were expected to have mastered the scientific material necessary to the care of patients, and to have psychologically reached the stage where it would take more than the sight of blood to make them pass out. Hence, for their last two years of study they were assigned to ward duty on the different services: medicine, surgery, obstetrics and gynecology, pediatrics, and psychiatry. In addition, there were periods of elective time that could be spent on many of the smaller services. The students took histories, performed physical examinations, and helped with their patients' ongoing medical care under the supervision of graduate physicians.

They also did a load of scut work. "Scut" is a word reputedly derived from the Greek term for excrement, and it was used in reference to the innumerable unpleasant little tasks which were, in most private hospitals, performed by non-medical workers. At The Vue, however, these jobs slid down the chain of command to the bottom, where they settled among the medical students and interns. Performing blood counts was scut, and so was wheeling patients to and from the X-ray Department. No less scutty was having to run the length of the hospital to Central Supply when the electrocardiograph machine ran out of paper in the middle of working up a patient.

The scut jobs at The Vue were endless, and medical students spent an inordinate amount of their time wondering how it came to pass that their tuition fee involved them in more hours of doing scut than making ward rounds with attending physicians. When they protested, they were patronizingly told that scut was, after all, also an L.E. (Bellevuese for "Learning Experience"), to which the students would usually react with an expletive that meant scut.

After four years of medical school, and having mastered the fundamentals of basic medical science and patient care, the student was permitted to put M.D. after his name, and was graduated into internship. Now the learning process began in earnest.

Although the intern was technically an employee of Bellevue Hospital (being paid a munificent $3,200 per year), he was part of the affiliated medical school teaching staff together with his more senior house officers—the residents and the staff of attending physicians. He learned from his superiors and he helped to teach the students beneath him.

Working on the wards and in the clinics all day, and taking calls through many of the nights, the intern was first on the firing line in the care of his patients. By doing what he could by himself, and by helping his seniors with more difficult tasks, his fund of knowledge and reservoir of confidence gradually increased. It is generally true that most doctors have learned more during their internship than during any other single year of their lives.

Upon completion of internship, the doctor became a resident physician. Residency consisted of a set number of years of training, during the course of which there was progressive assumption of more complex duties and greater responsibilities, all of which ultimately led to the doctor's capacity to function independently as a specialist in a particular field. The length of time spent in residency varied with the specialty, ranging from two years in pediatrics to seven or more years for some of the surgical sub-specialties. Residents supervised the work of interns and medical students, and they, in turn, were supervised by more senior residents and by attending physicians.

For all practical purposes, the chief residents on the various specialties were the kingpins of The Vue. In consultation with their attending physicians, they made the ultimate decisions regarding patient care, performed the most difficult operations, and generally kept watch over their entire services. When an intern or a junior resident blundered, the chief resident was held accountable. When all was going well on a service, that was merely to be expected. The buck definitely stopped on the chief's desk. After surviving that sort of a year, the graduating chiefs were ready for anything that practice had to offer.

The senior members of the teaching team were the attendings, of which there were two types. Part-time attendings were men and women in practice who wished to maintain a strong association with a medical school. Therefore they donated their time to help with the on-the-job training for the medical students and the house staff. The full-time attendings, on the other hand, were paid a salary by the school in return for which they taught at Bellevue, gave lectures to the pre-clinical students, and did research. Even at the attending physician level, the Bellevue fondness for hierarchism exerted itself: the attendings were placed at either the junior or the senior level.

At Bellevue, no service had anything good to say about any other service. According to the surgeons, the internists were a bunch of pusillanimous dudes, many of whom wore glasses, and were given to interminable arguments over picky, unimportant details of diagnosis or therapy, usually carried out while the patient was dying before their eyes. In return, the internists regarded the surgeons as mindless technicians, peculiar hybrids of butchers and tailors, who were happy only when they were up to their armpits in blood—someone else's blood, to be specific. Obstetricians and gynecologists either hated their mothers, enjoyed seduction, or were simply incapable of understanding anything more complicated than crotch plumbing. Pediatricians were afraid of adults. Urologists were animals, barely able to speak intelligible English. Dermatologists hated the sight of blood as much as surgeons loved it. And psychiatrists, of course, were nuttier than their patients.

Fortunately, behind all the name-calling was the obvious recognized fact that the services were interdependent in terms of their own survival, let alone that of the patients. That prevented the potential antagonisms from ever going beyond the banter stage.

The Bellevue patient-care system was centered around the Admitting Office. This was something of a misnomer, since much more than the mere admitting of patients was carried out there. The A.O. was the general receiving area where those seeking medical attention presented themselves and were sorted out and disposed of according to their particular needs. Doctors assigned to the Admitting Office looked over each new patient and then decided how he or she might best be served by the Bellevue setup.

Some patients came to the Admitting Office with problems that were neither acute nor serious: for example, a head cold. They did this in the hope of obtaining treatment more quickly than it could have been gotten in the Clinic, where a supplicant frequently sat on a wooden bench for four hours or longer before a doctor called his number. These patients generally were not pleased when they were given Clinic appointments for the next day and told they weren't sick enough to warrant care at the A.O.

Their protests were heated enough to melt the gelatin capsules in the medicine cabinets.

On the other hand, problems requiring immediate attention were handled on the spot. Lacerations were sutured, boils were lanced, asthmatic attacks were terminated, and strep throats were combated with shots of penicillin to the nether zones. In most cases, follow-up was achieved via the infamous Clinic.

Not all conditions could be handled in the Admitting Office, though. Patients requiring longer-term care were admitted to the inpatient service. When there was no need for continuous close attention or intensive care, the patients were sent to routine wards. However, a patient with a severe heart attack, major hemorrhaging, or an overdose of drugs would be wheeled to the Emergency Room. This was the equivalent of today's intensive-care unit, offering the best chance of survival to such critically ill people.

The performance of this human sorting function was often more then a little tough on the doctor's nervous system. No one wanted to give a Clinic appointment to a patient who would carry the appointment slip only as far as the front steps of the hospital, and then proceed to drop dead. On the other hand, every admission had to be considered with the utmost care. When a patient was admitted, an intern or a resident had to work up the individual, and that usually meant many hours of labor, involving a history, a physical examination, and laboratory scut. That was fine if the patient were truly sick, but God help the Admitting Office doctor who caused one of his buddies to be up all night with a crock. (A crock is a non-sick patient, a hypochondriac, a malingerer, or an hysteric. Most doctors are very unfond of them.) The A.O. physician often felt that whatever course of action he took, someone was going to bitch at him. Unfortunately, this perception was usually accurate.

Perhaps the best way to sum up Bellevue is to say that it was a crisis-oriented place. Most of the patients who came there for care were truly good and sick. Then, as now, poor people did not have much truck with preventive medicine, thereby usually giving the illness a generous head start before they dragged themselves in for care.

And where did these disease-ravaged persons go for help when the inevitable could be put off no longer? To an institution chronically short of critical equipment, nurses, and aides, whose physical facilities seemed to sag in response to the weight they were forced to bear, where interns less than a year out of medical school and often with no sleep the night before tried to cope with, understand, and adjust to a constant struggle of life-and-death proportions.

No wonder Bellevue was the setting for innumerable astonishing episodes of peculiar, eccentric, and downright zany behavior. Patients and staff alike were subjected to pressures capable of taxing minds beyond the limits of tolerance; and to survive in that unusual environment sometimes required behavior which, viewed dispassionately, would have to be classified as something other than normal. Try to keep this in mind if the view from The Vue seems a little distorted in spots.

1

Don't Go Away Mad

Once, when I told a young woman that I was working at Bellevue Hospital, she burst out with, "Oh, that must be just *fascinating*. That's where they send all the *real* nuts." I assumed that she was referring to the patients in the Bellevue Psychiatric Pavilion, but I did worry a bit. In any case, my new acquaintance rapidly followed up her emphatic declaration with a request that I tell her "all about it."

That, in fact, would have been a major project. The Bellevue psychiatry building, constructed in 1935, was already long outmoded by the time I went to work there. Its seven floors of wards were divided into facilities designed to provide care for inmates according to their degree of impairment. The most seriously disturbed patients were confined on the top floor; below them were the moderately ill. The remainder of the building was given over to the care of patients with less critical mental disorders and to outpatients. Parts of two of the floors were set aside as psychomedicine wards, for mental patients who also suffered from serious bodily illnesses.

The physical characteristics of the psych building did very little to enhance the moods of inmates suffering from depression. Any patient who was not depressed on admission, and was capable of relating to his environment, didn't take long to experience a whopping dejection of spirits. Windows were few in number, and those that did exist were covered with bars. The hallways were long, dark, and dirty. Wards were overcrowded, understaffed, filthy, and malodorous. The beds were crammed into every available alcove, one right next to the other. Patients were either sprawled on the beds or sat on wooden chairs, usually

1

clutching their belongings in paper bags, to guard against the otherwise inevitable theft. Too often, they simply stared into space; there was nothing else to do.

The wards for the most serious patients were genuine chambers of horrors. Shrieks, screams, and groans reverberated down the corridors in a never-ending cacophony. Here and there a patient stood motionless, perhaps with a stream of urine running down his leg to form a puddle at his feet. Others lay uncommunicative, apparently unaware of the feeding tubes which were keeping them alive.

The worst patients, those reduced to either animal or vegetable status by deficiency or aberration of mentality, passed the time by mutilating themselves or others at every opportunity, or by assuming a rigid fetus-like posture for weeks or months on end. Therapeutic psychiatry being as primitive as it was, all we could do for these people was to keep them fed, relatively clean, quiet, and as far from harm's way as possible. Had they been dogs or horses, we'd have shot them without a second thought. But they were human beings, so we gave them tranquilizers.

My first exposure to psychiatry at The Vue came during my second year of medical school. We had a series of weekly lecture-demonstrations at which the professors would describe the manifestations of the different psychiatric diseases, and would then interview illustrative cases before us. It looked very easy.

The doctor sat in a chair opposite the patient, a picture of calm assurance, asking question after question, and appearing not in the least disturbed when the patient gave a seemingly inappropriate answer. When that happened, the professor usually picked up on something the patient had said and quickly changed the direction of his inquiry, but he was never at a loss for something to say. He maintained, at all time, an attitude that bespoke thorough command of the situation; he was totally unflappable. I thought that psych was going to be a breeze.

When the third year came around, I was assigned to spend six weeks on the psychiatry service. I was in a group of eight medical students assigned to Dr. Samuel Rothstein. Dr. Rothstein was a large, handsome man in his mid-forties whose eyes exuded kindness and understanding. On the first morning, he took us to the ward, selected a patient, and began to talk with him. The patient was a hopeless schizophrenic and, in response to Dr. Rothstein's quiet but firm probing, told us all about the astonishing collection of disembodied voices and peculiar creatures which lived within the distorted confines of his mind. The performance sent shivers along the vertebral columns of the uninitiated, but there seemed to be no reason for trepidation or anxiety. It still looked very easy.

After Dr. Rothstein had dismissed the patient, he answered our questions. Then he told us he thought we were ready to try a psychiatric interview on our own. He handed each of us a piece of paper. Mine bore the name Robert Jackson. Dr. Rothstein told us that after we had interviewed and examined our patients, he'd discuss their problems with us. Buoyed by eagerness and enthusiasm, I went off in search of Mr. Jackson.

The ward nurse told me that Mr. Jackson usually hung out "over there." She pointed to the end of a long corridor. I thanked her and strutted away, chin high.

As I made my way along the corridor, I began to notice the figures alongside me. They were men of all ages, sizes, and shapes; all in the same general state of disrepair. Some were sitting or lying motionless; others rocked to and fro; and still others paced. A middle-aged man, wearing a hospital bathrobe and badly in need of a shave, came forward and clutched at my spotless white coat. As he did, I pulled away by reflex.

Suddenly I realized I was all by myself, and that I was not only going to have to interview one of these patients, but also perform a physical examination. All my confidence emulsified and floated out the nearest window, between the bars. My pace slowed perceptibly, and I almost tripped over an old man who was stretched out across the hallway.

I had no sooner recovered myself than he grabbed my pants leg and wouldn't let go. After I had pulled away, I went on past another fellow who was masturbating onto the immobile, staring schizophrenic next to him; and then I passed a codger who was holding his little paper bag of personal belongings in his left hand, while he used his right hand to direct his stream of urine against the wall. By the time I reached the end of the hallway, I was shaking. I saw a young man sitting there, staring out the window. In a voice about two octaves higher than my usual, I asked, "Mr. Jackson?"

Mr. Jackson turned very slowly, and then took about thirty seconds to glare at me. He was about twenty-five years old, and he had long, straight black hair, and the most angry, hating, hostile eyes I have ever seen. Going up another octave, I explained that I was Dr. Karp, and that I had come to interview him.

Silently he motioned me to sit down in the chair next to him. I thanked him, sat down, and gave my folder of papers a professional shuffle.

My mind was racing. I thought, My God, what happens if I ask this guy a wrong question and he gets pissed off at me? He'll kill me and drink my blood and leave me lying here and they'll never find me; they'll think I'm just another catatonic patient.

Finally I forced myself to be calm. I'm being silly, I thought. He won't hurt me. And I won't ask any wrong questions. I drew a couple of deep breaths and then noticed that all this time Mr. Jackson was staring at me with hostility in his eye and a sardonic little smile at the corners of his mouth.

I knew I had to start talking, and I drew in another breath. No hesitancy now, Karp. Show him who's boss.

"Well, Mr. Jackson," I said. "Why don't you tell my why you're here in the hospital?"

Mr. Jackson ran the fingers of his right hand through his hair. Then he looked up slowly and glared into my eyes.

"Well, Doc," he drawled, in a subtly mocking tone, "it's like this. The reason I'm here is that I think all the paranoids in the world are out to get me."

In the end, I managed to survive my interview with Mr. Jackson, but it took a bit of prodding by Dr. Rothstein to get me to see my second assigned patient. Fortunately, that encounter was considerably less traumatic, and after interviewing and examining a few more patients, I even managed to regain a part of my original confidence. One issue, though, continued to haunt me and make me uneasy: the claim by the patients that they had been railroaded to Bellevue. It seemed that every patient I interviewed, who was in any way capable of conversation, sooner or later informed me that he or she was at that moment talking to me only because an enemy had arranged for the patient to be involuntarily committed. The sole variation on the theme was in the nature of the enemy.

By far the most frequent committer of the innocent was the F.B.I. It seemed, however, that the Feds persecuted only the most blatantly psychotic inmates, and it was pretty easy to disregard such a complaint when the patient followed it up by pointing his finger at an uninhabited corner to show me the G-man who was still tailing him day and night. Less clear-cut were the situations involving supposed commitments because of the complaint of a spouse or another relative. Sometimes the hospital records bore out the basic truth of the complaint, sometimes not. In either event, as a group, the patients making this claim did not seem as strange as the F.B.I. bunch, and I experienced a good bit of difficulty in trying to sort out justified anger from paranoia.

What do you think when an enraged, but seemingly coherent man tells you that the cops dragged him off to The Vue because his wife claimed he had attacked her with a knife, but that in reality he had done no such thing. To make the situation thoroughly incomprehensible, a patient of this sort sometimes also said that his wife had been trying to get rid of him for some time, and that the first thing he was going to do upon his release was kill her. Such a guy was definitely more than a little dangerous, yes. But crazy? I could never tell. Every now and then, one of the less violently inclined "referrals" would eventually get out and promptly hire a lawyer in an attempt to squeeze a little monetary compensation out of the city.

No such patient caused me more confusion—and embarrassment—than Solomon Washington. Mr. Washington was one of the patients assigned to me during my third-year clerkship. He had been admitted late the previous night, and when I sat down to interview him, had not yet run the gamut of the residents. He was still quite willing to talk to a doctor. In fact, he was eager.

He was a huge black man, weighing well in excess of two hundred pounds, and stood six-four in his paper Bellevue slippers. His bearing was of extreme, perhaps excessive, dignity, which at times approached the Amos n' Andy burlesque style. But despite the physical resemblance and the similarity of mannerisms, Mr. Washington was no Andrew H. Brown. By his own account (which was very readily offered) he was a 1950 graduate of the University of Pennsylvania, with a major in economics.

"With that kind of background, what are you doing living on the Bowery?" I asked him.

"Please don't be so crass as to think that every resident of a Bowery flophouse is an ignorant, uneducated hobo," he answered. "The common denominator of Bowery existence is nothing more than lack of money. There are those of us who simply are down on their luck, you might say."

"I didn't think jobs were so hard to come by for economists," I said, my voice a bit snottier than was called for.

"Oh, true, very true indeed, my dear young fellow," said Mr.

Washington with all the haughtiness at his command. "You are quite right, if you're talking about *white* economists. But I'd like to see *you* in *my* skin for a little while, trying to get a job. Perhaps then you'd understand better. No, the unfortunate truth is that Negroes just aren't faring terribly well at the moment in the economics job markets."

Round one to Mr. Washington.

"Let's go on," I said hastily. "Why don't you tell me how you happened to end up at Bellevue." I smiled in what I hoped was an ingratiating manner.

"I'll be most happy to, if you'd like," he said. "Though I must say, it *is* a rather painful subject—literally painful, I might add." He rubbed a black-and-blue area under his left eye, as though for emphasis.

"I'd appreciate it," I said. "It'll help me understand your case better."

Mr. Washington shook his hand rapidly back and forth. "No problem at all," he said. "It's quite straightforward, really. Last night, at about three o'clock, I was standing on the corner of Third Avenue and Fourteenth Street when some young men—some young *white* men, to be specific—accosted me and asked whether I had a match. It happened that I didn't. You see, I don't smoke, and so don't usually have matches on my person. I told them I was sorry, whereupon they became rather abusive. They started to call me names, and—"

"What names did they call you?" I asked.

Mr. Washington rolled his eyes expressively. "Well, Doctor," he said. "They began with nigger, as perhaps you might have expected, and they . . . well, shall we say, they accused me of behavior that would have made Oedipus feel uncomfortable."

I fought to keep my face properly straight. I nodded soberly, and gave a professional um-hum. "What did you do?" I asked.

"Now, Doctor . . . uh . . . I'm sorry, what did you say your name was?"

"Karp."

"Oh yes, Dr. Karp. Certainly. As I was about to say, Dr. Karp, I'm not trained as a prize fighter. I'm not aggressive and I do all I can to avoid violence. I tried to walk away. But they didn't permit me to do that. They followed me, calling me those terrible names, and then one of them shoved me into the wall of a building while another one punched me in the stomach. At that point I decided that I had been forced to take a stand, so I hit the second fellow, the one who had punched me. When I did that, all of the miserable hoodlums jumped on me and started to beat me up. I fought back as well as I could, but I was definitely getting the worse of the affair when two policemen came by and broke up the fight. I couldn't have been more grateful, of course, and was about to thank my benefactors when one of the young men said, 'That nigger bum tried to get a quarter off us, and when we wouldn't give it to 'im he pulled a razor on us.' Before I could utter a single word of the truth in my defense, one of the policemen hit me with his billy club and knocked me unconscious. The next thing I knew, I was a guest in your establishment."

I talked to Mr. Washington for a while longer and could uncover no mental aberrations. There were no signs of psychosis: he did not seem to suffer from delusions or hallucinations. He was oriented as to time and place, knew who the President was, could count backward from one hundred by sevens, and could correctly explain the meanings of different proverbs. The longer we spoke, the more convinced I became that because Mr. Washington was black and penniless, he had indeed been railroaded to The Vue. I began to feel angry. Finally, I could think of no further questions to ask him, so I thanked him and explained that I was going to present his case to the doctor in charge.

Mr. Washington stood up and extended his hand, which I gripped. "Thank you very much, Dr. Karp," he said. "I do trust that you will attempt to effect my prompt release from this unjustified confinement."

I assured him emphatically that I was firmly in his corner, proceeded directly to the chart rack, pulled out his chart, and read the police report from the cops who had brought him in. It said that he had been drunk and abusive, but made no mention of his set-to with the gang of white youths. I ground my teeth loudly. Did they have to add falsification by omission to injustice?

Leaving a cloud of smoke to mark my spot, I sought out Dr. Rothstein and poured out the story in a torrent. Dr. Rothstein stood there quietly throughout my performance. When I finished, he asked, "What did the admitting resident have to say about him?"

I gulped. My righteous indignation had prevented me from looking past the police report. Together we went back to the chart rack and read the resident's writeup. It was concise and to the point. It said that Mr. Washington had reeked of the demon rum and that he hadn't been making much sense when he spoke. The resident's diagnosis was: acute alcoholic psychosis.

"That psych Admitting Office is a snakepit," I said hastily. "Maybe the resident read the police report but didn't have enough time to actually spend talking to Mr. Washington."

"That's possible," Dr. Rothstein said. "But I don't think it's very likely."

Neither did the rational part of my mind, but that entity had already been submerged in my emotions. "*You* come and talk to him," I urged. "You'll see he's no more crazy than we are."

Dr. Rothstein smiled and followed me to Mr. Washington. He listened as the patient told his story again, and then we walked away together.

"Well?" I asked as we moved out of earshot.

"I think he ought to stay for observation for another day or two," said Dr. Rothstein. He held up his hand to stop my howl of protest before it could start. "Tell you what," he continued. "I'd like you to check up on him periodically during the day. Then tonight, before you go home, leave your phone number and tell them to call you if there's any . . . change in his condition. Okay? Just be a little patient; I think you may learn something from this case."

Mr. Washington appeared to be fine all day, but when I stopped to say good-night to him, he seemed agitated. His hands shook as he tried to eat his dinner, and he couldn't seem to sit still in his chair. I asked what was wrong.

"If you were confined in a place like this," said Mr. Washington, in a bass whine, "I assure you, you'd feel nervous too."

I tried to reassure him, and told him to hold out till morning, at which time I'd again attempt to have him released.

At a quarter to one in the morning, my phone rang. The ward clerk told me to come right over, that Mr. Washington's condition had definitely changed.

My first reaction upon arriving at the ward was mixed disbelief and anger. Mr. Washington was strapped into a restraint bed, and he was struggling so fiercely that the whole apparatus was bouncing about on the floor. He was screaming unintelligible words and sentence fragments, and his finely measured speech had vanished. His vocabulary and dialect had become pure Bowery.

I leaned over him. "Mr. Washington, Mr. Washington," I shouted. "What's the matter? What have they done to you?" His eyes rolled uncontrollably. "Oooooh, no!" he wailed. "No, no, no, no, no! Ge'em oudda here, ge'em away." He brushed clumsily at the air in front of his face. Streams of sweat rolled off his forehead in every direction. A nurse walked up beside me. "First time you see a good case of the DT's?" she asked. "That's the delirium tremens, when they sees things an' hears things an' shakes all over." She shook her head and chuckled. "I just dunno. These ol' alkies, long as they keep drinkin' they're okay, but then they come in here an' go a day without no booze, they all get the DT's." She jabbed a needle into Mr. Washington's rump, emptied the syringeful of tranquilizer, and crooned, "Doncha worry now, honey, this's gonna make all them snakes 'n' elephants go 'way, hear?"

My ears began to burn. I could have killed Mr. Washington for hoodwinking me, and I would not have suffered a pang of remorse. Nor were my feelings mitigated the next morning when Dr. Rothstein asked me to tell the group about my patient, and then, with an arch smile, he asked me whether I had learned anything from the case.

Bellevue abounded in contrasts. Two years later, as an intern on the psychomedicine ward, I took care of Mr. Washington's opposite number. His name was Harold Bullock, and he even looked like Mr. Washington. Bullock was brought in one evening as a florid DTer, screaming and hallucinating, having been picked up on a midtown street. He was uncontrollable on admission, and it took four of us to get him into restraints. Only when we had sedated him was I able to examine him. I could find nothing of significance aside from his disorientation and a fever of 101°. There was no infectious explanation for the latter, and so I chalked it up to the joint effect of alcohol and agitation, and proceeded to treat him for his DT's.

On rounds the next day, Mr. Bullock was no better, but that wasn't unusual: attacks of DT's can last for days. However, his temperature was now 102.6°, and our resident, Dr. Ronnie Edelson, frowned as he took note of that. "Where's the fever coming from?" he asked me sharply.

I shrugged. "I guess it's just the DT's," I answered. "His chest is clear; there's no urinary tract infection; no abscesses on him; liver's not enlarged. It must be a metabolic fever."

Ronnie looked back at Mr. Bullock, and pulled thoughtfully at his chin. Then he leaned over, put his hand under the patient's head, and lifted. Mr. Bullock's entire body rose off the bed. I noticed a very unpleasant sinking sensation in the pit of my stomach.

"*Schmuck!*" said Ronnie, in a withering tone. "This guy's neck is as rigid as a board. He's got meningitis. Plenty of alkies do, y'know. Get a hold of an LP tray and do a spinal tap, fast."

Less than ten minutes later I had a needle in Mr. Bullock's back. I expected to see pure pus come out of it, but when I removed the stylet, to my amazement, out flowed crystal-clear fluid. I collected a sample of it, took it to the lab, and analyzed it. Then I went looking for Ronnie.

"I don't know why he's so stiff," I said, "but one thing he *hasn't* got is meningitis. His fluid's perfectly benign. No bacteria in it, no pus cells—"

"Was it under increased pressure?"

"High normal. But not elevated."

Ronnie shook his head. "With a neck like that he's got to have meningitis," he said. "Did you send a sample for culture?"

"I asked them to check for every bacterium I could think of."

"Did you ask for fungal cultures too?"

"Fungi?" I wrinkled my forehead. "That's reaching pretty far out, isn't it?"

"Did you?"

"No, I didn't. I really didn't think . . ."

"No, that's right. You didn't think," said Ronnie, thoroughly exasperated. "I'll only forgive you because it's early in the internship year. Listen. One thing you've got to learn is that Bellevue is a far-out place, and you've got to think of far-out diseases here. When you work at a nice, respectable hospital like Beth Israel, and you hear hoofbeats, you can pretty much count on seeing horses. But at The Vue, it's more likely to be zebras—or even unicorns. So you go back and tell the lab to do fungal cultures on that spinal fluid. Get an India ink prep too."

"What the hell's an India ink prep?" I asked.

"It's for a fungus called cryptococcus," said Ronnie. "You can read about it; it's spread by airborne dissemination of particles of bird shit. You mix India ink on a slide with the spinal fluid, and the ink stains the cryptococcus so it shows up under the microscope."

I snickered, and then took a look at Ronnie's face. "All right, all right," I mumbled. "I'll get it all. Maybe he raises pigeons or something."

Ronnie grinned. "*Now* you're starting to think," he said. "And while we're waiting for the results, you'd better start him off on penicillin and a broad-spectrum antibiotic. That'll cover most of the bacteria, and we'll keep after the lab for a quick culture result."

I did what Ronnie wanted, and then spent the rest of the day chasing one problem after another. About five o'clock, I was sitting at the charting desk drinking a bottle of soda when the phone rang. The clerk answered it and then waved the receiver in my direction. "Lab callin', Dr. Karp," she said.

I took the phone and said hello. The voice at the other end asked whether I was Dr. Karp; I assured it I was.

"You ordered an India ink prep on a patient Bullock?"

"Yep. What about it?"

"What's about it is that it's positive! Damn slide was crawling with cryptococcus! Dr. McKenzie here in the lab says he's never seen so many bugs on a slide."

I whispered a thank-you, hung up the phone, and penitently went looking for Ronnie Edelson. He looked annoyed as I gave him the report. "That's not something you ought to be joking about," he said. "What if I took you seriously?"

"You'd better take me seriously," I answered. "That stupid India ink prep was as positive as it could be. I'm not kidding."

"You're kidding," said Ronnie. He looked closely at me. "No, I don't think you are," he said slowly. Then he started to laugh.

"Now do you believe in unicorns?" he asked.

We treated our unicorn with intravenous infusions of amphotericin B, the only antibiotic effective against cryptococcus, and a drug so toxic that it can cause livers and kidneys to rot. Every time I infused it, it produced such a severe reaction in the vein that the blood vessel was thereafter useless. Since it took two months to cure Mr. Bullock, I wiped out virtually every vein on his body except the one running on top of his penis. A couple of times near the end of his treatment, even that one was in danger.

Far from being an alcoholic, Mr. Bullock turned out to be a very solid citizen who had been employed in a midtown office. On investigation, we learned that his desk had been located right next to the air conditioner, and that a flock of pigeons had been in the habit of dropping their loads on the outside window ledge. The air conditioner, subsequently, had blown in a pure culture of cryptococcus for Mr. Bullock to inhale. He had been complaining of headaches, nausea, and dizziness for a few days before the cops found him on the street.

When he regained his right mind, we offered to transfer him to the general medical service, out of the psych building, but he refused. "You knew what was wrong with me," he said, "and I figure you saved my life. I don't want anyone else treating me." So Mr. Bullock cheerfully spent two months locked in the psychomedicine ward. He was not in the least unhappy about having been railroaded.

The multiple problems we encountered in trying to treat psychotic patients with medical illnesses are illustrated in the case of Mr. James St. Peter. James was admitted to the psychomedicine ward one night during the first week of my internship. He was suffering from pneumonia, and had been sent to psych because of his obvious dementia. I couldn't be certain whether he was retarded, schizophrenic, or both. Some people are doubly blessed. In any case, all he did was babble incoherently at people or objects that he either was hallucinating or pretending to see. He was an emaciated, eighty-pound, totally bald, black man. As he lay in his bed behind the safety rails, he demonstrated terrible anxiety and apprehension. His eyes almost popped out of his head as he continually looked about, glancing here and there, and addressing questions and answers to invisible companions. Now and then he managed to answer a question that I put to him before he floated away again into the other world.

We treated his pneumonia with antibiotics, and although his condition improved, even when his fever broke he was no less delirious. He had been in the hospital for a couple of days when a faculty psychiatrist came by to make rounds with us. When he reached James's bed, he asked the little man several questions, but James was too busy conversing with the spirit world to pay the Shrink any mind. Finally, the psychiatrist leaned over the bed rail and, nose to nose with the patient, boomed out, "James, now tell me: Did you ever do anything bad—like robbing a liquor store?"

The little fellow came back to what we call reality. He looked up in panic at the psychiatrist, his eyes protruding far in front of his face, and stammered, "N-n-n-no-suh. Hain't nevuh did dat. B-b-b-but—St. Peter James—St. Peter James—he done it." Then he went back to play with his friends.

The psychiatrist looked at the name at the foot of the bed. It read, James St. Peter, the same as on the admission slip. "Aha," exclaimed our Freud image. "That's classic." He smiled smugly. We all looked at each other, and finally the resident decided to swallow his pride in the interest of knowledge. "Classic for what, sir?" he asked.

"Why, for schizophrenia! That's what they always do. Not only do they assume another personality, but they give the other personality the inverted form of their own name. That way, it symbolizes that the assumed personality—who they usually perceive as evil—is the opposite of what they are themselves." He smiled magnanimously at the group. All of us swine nodded and tucked the pearl away for future use.

The psychiatrist was so enthusiastic that over the next couple of days he brought several groups to our ward to see the classic patient. Psychiatric colleagues, residents, and medical students all got to hear, "St. Peter James—St. Peter James—he done it."

James's pneumonia was responding so well that we were already thinking about which nursing home we could send him to when, one afternoon, the nurse called to tell us that James St. Peter's blood pressure was unobtainable. We found him cold and clammy; a physical examination and an X-ray showed us that a lung abscess, previously hidden by the pneumonia, had ruptured and sent the patient into shock. This bacterial shock, even now a terribly serious problem, was at that time, for all practical purposes, a death sentence. But we tried. We pumped into James every medication we thought might have a chance of helping him, but he continued to deteriorate. So, I decided we'd better call the next of kin. I asked the nurse whether any such were listed for the patient. She checked the chart and hollered back, "Yeah, Dr. Karp, he's got a brother, William."

"Call him," I said. "Tell him to come to the hospital right away, and I'll talk to him." I shuddered at the thought of having to explain a dying James St. Peter to a physically healthy version.

About half an hour later there was a pounding on the locked door. The nurse went to open it. In raced a gigantic, muscular man about two and a half times the size of my patient. Now I really shuddered. I looked around, but there were no other doors on the ward. I was stuck. I figured I'd better get it over with, so I introduced myself to the weeping man and explained why I had called him here. After a few minutes of talking to him, I realized that he was sound—not only of body, but of mind as well. Furthermore, he was very upset about his brother, and begged to be allowed to see him before he died; so we went together into James's room.

William leaned over the bed and called, "Hey, buddy, it's me— William—hey, look up at me." But James was going to spend his last moments with his private friends, and he didn't even cast his brother a glance.

William and I walked away from the bed. He seemed a bit more composed now, and drew a sigh. "I've been figuring something like this was gonna happen for a while," he said. "I want to thank you for taking care of him and trying to help."

The speech was made with tremendous sincerity and dignity. In reply, I stuttered a little, and finally managed to say, "Thank you, Mr. St. Peter."

The man turned and looked down at me in bewilderment. "No, no," he said. "You've got it wrong. My brother is St. Peter."

Now I was bewildered. "But . . . aren't you both St. Peter? He's James St. Peter, and you're Will—"

"Oh, I see," he interrupted. "No, he's not James St. Peter. His name is St. Peter James. I'm William James. You've got it backwards." He smiled tolerantly at me.

I flushed and pawed at the floor with my right toes.

"Matter of fact," continued William James, "his name is really Allen St. Peter James. But he always went by his middle name." Then he paused a moment and added, "You people here seem kind of mixed up."

In retrospect, I think Mr. James was right. But it should be kept in mind that the Bellevue Psychiatric Pavilion was not a place where wealthy neurotics came to stretch out on a couch at fifty dollars a half hour. The clientele were genuine end-of-the-roaders, and they descended in hordes on an understaffed, underequipped hospital whose primary asset was the grittiness of its personnel. If this staff did, indeed, become a little mixed up now and again, it was both understandable and forgivable.

2

It's Hard to Get Good Help Nowadays

Understaffing was a perpetual major problem at The Vue. It's true that there was never a shortage of interns and residents, but there never was enough of anyone else. The house staff might have been persuaded to work at The Vue because of the tremendous educational potential, but this hardly constituted an inducement to nurses, aides, orderlies, elevator operators, messengers, or laundry workers. To them, The Vue was just a big filthy, depressing place, where the pay was lousy, the hours long, and where it was easily possible to contract a dreadful disease without even having gotten any pleasure out of it.

A large proportion of the ancillary help were dedicated people. They had to be. A nurse might come in to work on the midnight-to-eight shift and find herself responsible for covering anywhere from four to eight wards. She'd barely have time to finish passing out one round of medication before it was time to repeat the whole process. And as for playing the Nightingale bit, she just had to forget that ambition. On the night shift at The Vue, there was no time to comfort the sick or reassure the dying. It was a victory simply to keep the Spartan inhabitants properly medicated in the hope that perhaps some of them might get better.

There were also none of the pleasant little services that private hospitals provide to make the lives of interns and residents more bearable. Smiling young women did not come around each morning and draw the bloods for testing; unshaved interns did. Interns also, personally, performed blood counts. When they had finished doing that, they filled out X-ray requests, and hand-delivered them to the X-ray department. And when X-ray called for Mr. Jackson to come down for his barium enema, an intern

15

would wheel him down, lift him onto the table, wait while the procedure was being done, lift him off, and take him back upstairs. By that time, the electrocardiograph machine might have run out of paper, and someone would have to hotfoot it over to Central Supply for some more. Guess who was the messenger?

True, there were some volunteers at The Vue, and they did some very nice things, like passing out books and toys to the clientele, or helping a paralyzed stroke victim do his exercises so he might regain some function in a limp arm or leg. Whatever human touch was offered at that place was due in large measure to the volunteers. But after he's been up all night, what does an intern care for the human touch? All he wants is a slave or a magician to make the scut work vanish.

I had one. I'm not certain whether she was slave or magician, but she got the job done. She was my wife, Myra, and she had to be the greatest volunteer in the history of The Vue. We once figured out that if the City of New York had paid her for the work she did, Gotham would have faced bankruptcy several years sooner.

Myra's unofficial career began one night during the autumn of my internship year. She had come to join me for dinner at the doctor's dining room, the gourmet establishment in the Bellevue basement where free meals were served to all house physicians. Since house physicians wore white jackets with the emblem, CITY OF NEW YORK, DEP'T OF HOSPITALS on the sleeve, interns' wives simply put on their husbands' extra jackets and walked in past Miz Matthews, the gigantic assistant dietician who used to station herself at the doorway to prevent any medical students or other ringers from cadging dinners.

It was a slow night. The weather hadn't yet turned cold enough to trigger epidemics of pneumonia and chilblains on the Bowery. We had finished up the ward work before supper, and at the moment there was nothing to do. So we sat and talked over second helpings of dessert, savoring the luxury of indolence far more than the food.

After a while I realized that the day's laboratory reports must have arrived back on the ward. It was the intern's job not only to review them, but to paste the slips into the charts as well. When I mentioned the lab slips, Myra picked up her pocketbook and made ready to leave.

"Wait a minute," I said. "There's nothing going on. Why don't you come up to the ward and keep me company while I do the slips?"

Myra looked uncertain.

"There's no problem," I continued. "No one's going to bother you, but if it makes you feel better, just leave the white coat on. You'll look like a med student."

Myra thought for a moment. "Okay," she said. "Guess it's better than sitting around the apartment."

We went upstairs. I checked through the pile of reports and then began to paste them into their owners' charts. Myra watched for a few minutes and then quickly grabbed half the pile of slips that were left. I looked up.

"No reason for me to just twiddle my thumbs," she said. "I don't think it takes any special training to stick these things into the charts."

We finished the lab slips in half the time it usually took me to do them alone, and a wonderful idea began to germinate in my cerebrum. "Come on," I said. "Let's go up to the lab and I'll show you how to do an admission blood-workup."

Myra protested that she couldn't possibly do that.

"Sure you can," I said. "They're the exact same tests that you learned in the human biology course you took in college. I'll just have to brush you up a little."

The lab was always an ungodly mess, and we had no trouble finding the remains of a tube of blood that some intern had left lying around earlier that day. Myra watched me perform a hemoglobin concentration, a hematocrit, and a white-cell count and differential examination.

"They really are just the same," she mused.

"I told you. Here. You try it." She did, and I checked her out. She was right on target. My joy knew no bounds.

By the time we returned to the ward, my little idea was ready to bear fruit. In our absence, a new patient had been wheeled up for me. The slip from the Admitting Office read, "ASHD, early CHF." This meant "arteriosclerotic heart disease, with early congestive heart failure." The patient attached to the note was a gentle, little, seventy-year-old man from the Lower East Side, and his swollen legs, pulsating neck veins, and rapid respirations all attested to his cardiac decompensation. I grabbed a needle and a syringe, and drew a blood sample from him.

Myra read my intentions accurately. She held out her hand and I gave her the tube of blood. She recoiled slightly. "It's . . . it's still warm," she said, her tone reflecting considerable dubiety and more than a passing wave of nausea.

"Hot from the vein," I said. "Now, you can do the blood tests while I take his history and examine him."

Myra gripped the tube more firmly. "All right, foxy husband," she said with a grin. "It's still better than sitting around the apartment while you're here."

"For me that goes double," I replied. She started off toward the lab as I wheeled the wheezing patient into the examining room and went to work.

By the time Myra returned, I had completed the history and the physical examination and had done an electrocardiogram to be as sure as I could that the episode of heart failure had not been triggered by a heart attack. Myra gave me the results of the lab work, and I entered them into the chart. Then, while I wrote up my conclusions, she left for X-ray with my charge, and returned with the views of his chest just as I was finishing up my notes. All I had to do was read the films and start the little man on therapy. My wife had saved me a good hour of scut work. An hour! More precious than platinum or petroleum to an intern! I had found El Dorado, and my euphoria was boundless.

Within days I was the envy of every other intern at The Vue. Sticking to her claim that it was better than sitting home alone, Myra would arrive around dinnertime on most of my nights on call. Miz Matthews soon was greeting her like one of the regulars, which, of course, was what she had become. After supper, we'd go up to the ward and take care of the lab slips and any necessary blood tests and urinalyses. New admissions now seemed like duck soup, and if nothing else was going on, I'd catch up on my chart reviews while Myra would give the nurse a hand by doing general aide's work. She drew the line at emptying bedpans, though. That, she said, was not better than sitting home alone.

When I finished my internship year and moved into the first year of residency training in obstetrics, my unofficial associate came along with me. We rapidly discovered that obstetrics was not only more to my taste, it was also more to my wife's taste. She delighted in the quick-paced excitement of the labor and delivery suite, where every blood count and every trip to X-ray was an emergency. Furthermore, she was able to acquire some new skills beyond doing lab work and running off to X-ray. Three delivery rooms were operating at full capacity, but with only one nurse, and occasionally an aide, to keep things going. Keeping things going involved setting out drapes and instruments, handing sutures and other necessary equipment to the doctors, weighing, footprinting, and wrapping up the newborn babies, and then cleaning the rooms for the next round of deliveries. Myra learned to do it all, and the nurses were as ecstatic as I was.

Not everyone shared our enthusiasm, however. One of the senior residents complained endlessly to me that it was not proper for my wife to be there. No, he did not mean to imply that she was interfering with my concentration; and, yes, he did have to admit, she seemed to be serving a useful function. But nonetheless, he just thought that a resident's wife shouldn't be in the hospital when her husband was on call.

"Suppose my wife were a doctor too?" I asked him one night in exasperation. "Would she have to take her residency in another hospital so we wouldn't be on call together?"

"Of course not," the senior resident answered with hesitation. "That would be different." But just how it would be different he could never quite explain. So Myra kept coming to The Vue, and he kept bitching about it.

The matter was finally settled one night when one of our patients suffered a severe laceration at delivery. Blood poured from the woman's vagina so that the floor beneath the table looked like the Red Sea. The senior resident and I worked frantically to suture the hemorrhaging gash while the only other available resident pumped fluid and blood into the patient's arm.

"What's her hematocrit?" shouted the senior resident.

"I don't know," the pumping resident called back. "I drew a tube for it, but I can't leave off here long enough to run the thing."

In one breath, the senior resident managed to take both the names of the Lord and Savior in vain. "Get a hold of somebody who can do that hematocrit," he bellowed at no one in particular.

Without saying a word, Myra got up off the stool in the corner from where she had been watching the commotion. She took the tube of blood from the resident, and walked rapidly out of the delivery room. In a few minutes she was back.

"Hematocrit's 31," she said loudly.

"That's a low blood count for someone who's doing all this bleeding," the senior resident yelled. "Pump in that blood faster."

The other resident pumped faster, the senior resident and I sutured faster, and in a few minutes we achieved satisfactory hemostasis. The emergency was over.

I have to give the senior resident credit. As he peeled off his gloves he thanked Myra politely, and from that time on never failed to greet her warmly whenever he came up to labor and delivery and found her there. Myra had become one of the boys.

As such, she discovered even greater worlds to conquer. Blood counts were okay, and setting up rooms was fine, but nothing was really quite as fascinating as the deliveries themselves. Myra watched and listened, and before long was a fully qualified sidewalk midwife. She learned that there's no great trick to doing a routine delivery. The mother actually pushes the baby out, and the major responsibility of the attendant is to control the process, guiding the child out slowly and smoothly so that neither the baby's head nor the mother's bottom is damaged by a precipitous delivery.

Every three weeks a new batch of medical students came to the labor room, and they were assigned to patients in rotation. The residents helped them as much as they could, but there were too many laboring women and too few residents. Therefore, before they could learn the ropes, many students were forced to stand by in hysterical horror as their patients unceremoniously pushed out their newborns into their excrement-laden beds. *Inter urinam et faeces nascimur.*

One evening, as I was in the process of doing a forceps delivery, a first-night student flew into the room, his eyes wild with fear. "Come quick, Dr. Karp," he croaked, "The head's gonna come out."

"I can't stop in the middle of this one," I told him. "Go back and do the best you can from what you've read in the textbook, and I'll be there as soon as possible."

The poor guy shot out of the delivery room and into the hallway, where he ran directly into Myra. She had finished setting up one of the other delivery rooms, and was coming back to watch the forceps operation. The student had no idea who she was, but she must have looked as though she knew her way around the suite, because he grabbed her desperately and pleaded, "Do you know how to deliver a baby?"

Myra had seen enough frantic new students to be able to figure out what was happening. "Let's get back to your lady," she said coolly. "I'll help you out." And as they walked away I heard her say, "Now, the only thing you've really got to remember is just to keep it slow and smooth."

As they got to the labor room, they could see that the baby's head was very much in the process of coming out. "Put on your gloves," said Myra. "Now, put your right hand here, and your left hand there. That's it." She guided the student through the entire delivery, and when I checked the patient afterward I could find nary a tear.

"You didn't expect one, did you?" demanded my wife.

"Hell, no," I answered. "I figured you guys were at least as good as a couple of cab drivers."

"That's really fun," Myra said. "*I'd* like to be able to do it. Almost makes me want to apply to medical school."

I shuddered.

Before long the routine deliveries began to lose their challenge, and Myra moved on to bigger and better ones. She stood by as twins were being born, and watched fascinated as we delivered breech babies. The more unusual the procedure, the more my wife enjoyed it. She failed to get in on a caesarean section only because these patients had to be wheeled across a rooftop to get to the operating room halfway across the hospital, and in the general fuss and confusion Myra was concerned that she might really be in the way. But she saw every other manner of delivering a baby.

Well, almost every other manner. Sometimes a baby's head will be facing the wrong way in the birth canal, and the delivery can't be accomplished until it turns or is turned. In cases where spontaneous rotation fails to take place, a special forceps, designed by the Swedish obstetrician Kielland, can be used. But for some reason Kielland rotations were never performed while Myra was around. One night she even waited until three in the morning while a likely candidate labored, but at the very last minute the head rotated spontaneously. Myra muttered her way back to our apartment, convinced that the ghost of Dr. Kielland did not believe that wives of residents should be on delivery suites.

When the last week in June arrived, Myra knew that her days as obstetricians' helper had just about ended. Not only would I be leaving The Vue on July 1 to spend two years defending my country by delivering Navy wives, but she herself was nine months' pregnant. Very soon there would be valid reason for her to sit home at night. But while she could, she waddled around labor and delivery at The Vue, savoring every last minute of it.

The next-to-last night was a horror. No medical students were on call, there being a weekend's hiatus between groups. So, naturally, we were bombed with patients. I ran from one delivery room to the next just as quickly as the nurse and Myra could set them up and wheel the patients in. For every woman I delivered, another one was admitted. By midnight the hallway was lined on both sides with laboring and delivered patients, all mixed together. There wasn't even enough time to sort them out, let alone put them into labor rooms and post-partum ward beds.

I was as alone as I could possibly be; the senior resident and the chief resident had gone across the roof with a bleeding woman who needed an emergency caesarean section. There were no other doctors to give a hand. At that point, the tuberculosis ward called to tell me that one of their inmates had gone into labor.

I felt dizzy. It seemed that in one night I was fated to deliver every woman in New York City between the ages of fifteen and forty-four. I told the chest people to put a mask on their patient and send her over. She arrived a few minutes later, very much in labor. We found a spot for her against the wall.

Half an hour later, I was working with a patient in Delivery Room Two when Myra stuck her head in to announce that our tuberculous transfer was ready to have her baby. "Take her into Room One," I yelled, gesturing with my head. "I'll get there as soon as I can."

I delivered and sutured at double time, ripped off my gown and gloves, and ran toward Delivery Room One. As I got to the door, I heard the unmistakable howl of a newborn infant. "God damn!" I muttered. "Too late."

I walked into the room and froze in disbelief. The woman was up in the delivery position, and the baby was wrapped in a blanket and lying in the bassinet near the window. Between the patient's legs was my rotund wife in the process of catching the placenta in a basin as the woman pushed it out of her vagina.

"What are you doing?" I whispered.

Myra jumped as though goosed. "Oh, it's you," she said, her voice just a bit shakier than usual. I noticed that her hands were shaking too. "What the hell does it look like I'm doing?"

"But why you? Why didn't you get help?"

"Who from?" Myra snapped. "The other guys are still doing that section, and you were in the middle of your delivery. After I told you she was ready, I put her up in the stirrups and washed her so you'd be able to just run in and deliver her. But she didn't wait. She started to push the kid out; all I did was keep it slow and smooth. Thank God, the baby was in good shape. I put it in the bassinet, head down, and then I came back and caught the placenta when it fell out of her. I figured that was better than just standing there and letting her deliver with no help at all."

It all struck me as logical, but not quite kosher. "Why didn't you call Mrs. White?" I asked, simultaneously wondering where the nurse was.

As if for answer, Myra pointed toward Delivery Room Three. "Are you kidding?" she said with a little laugh. "She can't do two at a time either."

The dialogue was brought to an abrupt conclusion by a piercing shriek from the hallway. I ran out to find the inhabitant of one of the stretchers with her knees pulled up to her chest, alternately screaming hysterically and grunting like an eighty-year-old who hasn't had a bowel movement for a month. As I charged over, she grabbed me by the arm and shook me so that my teeth rattled. "Helpa me, helpa me," she implored wildly.

Simultaneously trying to free myself from her grasp and pull back the twisted sheet from her abdomen, I finally managed to get the baby, which was lying between her legs, almost totally immersed in a puddle of amniotic fluid. As I pulled the infant out by his feet, he gurgled, choked, and turned even bluer than he had been to start with. Since he was still attached by the umbilical cord, my mobility was severely limited. "Get me an emergency tray!" I howled at the top of my lungs. "Quick!"

Almost before the echoes had died down in the hallway, both Myra and Mrs. White were standing there, each holding an emergency delivery kit. I took one—I'm still not sure which—cut the baby free from his mother, and I sucked out what looked like a gallon of amniotic fluid from his nose, throat, and chest. To my immense relief, the kid turned pink, and let out a properly enraged howl.

After all the babies had been wrapped and sent to the nursery and their mothers had been taken down from the delivery stirrups, I slumped into the nearest chair. "Gawd," I mumbled. "What next?"

Another shriek from the hallway cut through the air. Simultaneously, I heard Mrs. White's always-calm voice: "Dr. Karp, come quick."

I got up running.

A deficiency of ancillary personnel is, of course, a relative matter, and since the early 1960's the situation at The Vue has been

ameliorated to some extent by medical insurance plans. Because
so many people are now covered by insurance, enabling them to
seek care from private doctors who practice at private hospitals,
smaller numbers of patients come to The Vue (and other city- and
county-supported institutions), and it is, therefore, easier to keep
up with them.

But now with New York City's desperate financial problems, it
can be predicted that the other part of the equation will also
diminish, and that there will be fewer nurses, aides, and messengers employed at The Vue in the years to come. My humble
suggestion to meet this crisis is straighforward: when internship
and residency candidates are interviewed for positions, talk to
their wives and girlfriends (or husbands and boyfriends) as well. A
newly created volunteer position of house-staff helper would
improve both the efficiency and the morale of the doctors at The
Vue, to say nothing of patient care. I'll testify to that at firsthand.

By the way, there's an epilogue to the story of Myra's Bellevue
career. Eight days after she left the hospital for the last time, she
entered University Hospital, right next door, to give birth to our
son. When the moment arrived, it was discovered that the mirror
which allowed women to watch their own deliveries was out of
whack; the screw holding the adjustment mechanism was loose so
the mirror couldn't be properly positioned. All obstetrics ceased
while a screwdriver was located, the offending screw tightened,
and the mirror adjusted to give Myra an unimpaired view of her
nether regions. Only then did the obstetrician apply the forceps,
turn the baby, and extract him.

"Was it really worth it, having everyone running after screw-
drivers like that?" I whispered to Myra as the obstetrician was
removing the placenta.

"Darn right it was," she said emphatically. "I finally got to see a
Kielland rotation."

3

Of Bums and Camel Drivers

The Bowery is the section of New York City which centers on Third Avenue below Fourteenth Street. During the late nineteenth century, it was the fashionable dining and theater area of the city, but that didn't last long. Before 1900, the place had already acquired a reputation as a locality where a citizen stood a pretty good chance of having his phrenology redesigned with a blunt instrument, and his wallet liberated. From that point, it was no time at all until the Bowery became New York's Skid Row, a collection of sleazy flophouses and greasy lunchstands where the sidewalks were littered with newspaper pages, broken bottles, nasopharyngeal oysters, and puddles of vomit. Thus it has remained to the present, inhabited by men (and occasionally women) who wander through the streets in alcoholic fogs, usually alert only to the likelihood that the next guy to nudge them in the ribs and say hello will be the skinny fellow in the black cape with the grinning face.

Such were the Bowery Bums, perhaps the principal customers of The Vue in the early 1960's. Their needs were many and varied, which was not terribly surprising. Basically, they were a bunch of guys who spent most of their time in the great outdoors, all year long.

In the summer, they had relatively few problems. The wards at The Vue were quiet, and the new house staff had time to learn their way around the hospital. Occasionally, one of the bums would be brought in with assorted fractures after having been hit by a car, but generally, things were peaceful.

By October, the leaves and the bums began to fall. An open doorway for a bed, and a newspaper for a cover, did not offer much protection from the New York winter winds and the cold, and the Bellevue ward population began to increase. By December, the natural elements and a diet of occasional bottles of Thunderbird wine combined to produce a full house at The Vue. In January, when even the healthy ones couldn't take it anymore, we were filled to capacity and we put 'em in the hallways, on the rafters, two to a bed, or anything else we could think of. This continued till March, when it began to let up a bit. By late May, Bellevue was quiet again, permitting the old hands among the house staff to finish up in peace. Then the new doctors reported in July, and the whole thing came full cycle.

I never could figure out why the bums stayed in New York for the winter. Birds went south. Golf caddies I knew when I was a boy in New Jersey would migrate to Florida in late September, spend the winter on the Sunshine State links, and then would appear back in New Jersey the next March all suntanned and hearty-looking, ready for another season. So why in God's name did the Bowery Bums have such an attachment to Third Avenue below Fourteenth Street? Why weren't the autumn streets filled with vast flocks of them crossing the Hudson to catch the freights as they rolled across the Jersey meadows?

Once I got curious enough to ask one of my patients this question. He considered the situation, and then shrugged and said, "Dunno. Never thought about it much."

I figured that pretty much answered the question. When you hit the Bowery, you've hit bottom; there's just nowhere else to go. You have no future and no hope; you're just marking time and waiting. When you hurt enough, you try, somehow, to make it stop. Total numbness is the *ultima thule*.

And so, the annual parade of infected lungs and rotten livers went on making their way to The Vue. The individual faces were familiar for a time, but for most of them it was a pretty short career. Attrition was high among the old-timers, and their places were rapidly assumed by the new arrivals. Youth must be served. The Bowery is a tough world.

One day during my internship, they wheeled in a guy for me to take care of. He was about forty, with wiry, gray hair and beautiful yellow skin. He wasn't Oriental though; it was his liver. He was out cold with hepatic failure. I figured that his liver must have been about the size of my pinky and have had both the appearance and the functional capacity of a piece of shoe leather. I really thought he had had it.

The nurse and I began to take off his clothes. As we did, dollar bills spilled out of his pockets and his underwear and scattered all over the bed. I seriously considered proctoscoping him. We gathered up the greenbacks and put them into an envelope with his name on it. Then we started him on treatment. I didn't think it would do any good, but he fooled me and began to recover. As the days passed, his skin color lightened and he even began to become responsive. Finally he reached the point where we could talk to him and expect to get a reasonable answer. So I asked him where he had gotten all that money. He must have forgotten about it till that moment, because he suddenly looked panicky and clutched at his pajama pockets. I assured him that the dough was in the hospital safe with his name on it. "I'm just curious where you got all that money," I said. "To be honest, you just don't look like a guy who'd have over a hundred bucks in his pockets. But you don't have to tell me if you don't want to."

The guy grinned at me. (Why did all Bowery Bums have only three widely separated teeth in their mouths?) "Don't mind at all. Gimme a cigarette, 'n' I'll tell yuh."

I didn't have any cigarettes, so I persuaded the bum in the next bed that it would be an act of charity and, in addition, he might learn how to get rich too. My patient lit up and began to talk. "I made it washin' car windows," he said. I guess I must have looked at him a little blankly, because he hastily added, "Y'know, down onna Bowery. When the cars stop fer red lights, I run out inna street 'n' wipe off the windas. Then I put out m' hand."

Now I understood. When you stop your car for a red light as you drive down the Bowery, these guys fly in swarms off the curbstones. They charge over, make a few passes at your windshield with a cruddy old rag, and then present themselves at your window, palm up. I myself had never paid one of these characters, first, because all they ever did was to streak the dirt across the windshield so that the visibility was worse than ever, and second, because I just plain resented having the bite put on me in that manner. So I told my patient that I couldn't imagine how he had made all that money at his occupation.

"Y'd be s'prized, Doc," he said. "I us'ally make 'bout forty bucks a day."

"Come on. That's a lot of windows."

"There's lotsa cars on the Bow'ry, Doc. Y'av'rage 'bout a quarter apiece, that's own'y a hunnert-sixty cars a day. Takes jus' a few hours, us'ally. Then I got the resta the day t' spend it on drinks fer me 'n' m' frien's." He dragged on the cigarette, and then continued, "B'sides, some guys even give a dollar."

"What about the people who don't give you anything?" I asked.

He smiled fiendishly. "Oh, I take care a' them guys."

I began to feel a little nervous.

He leaned over and stage-whispered at me, "Y'see what I do, Doc. I hang onna th' car, 'n' if the guy don' gimme nuthin, soon's 'e starts up, I grab m' foot 'n' yell, an' then I holler, 'I gotcher license number.' Y' be s'prised, Doc. Some guys gimme five bucks then. Serves the basstids right, too. I'd a been glad t' settle fer a quarter."

Maybe I ought to have been ashamed of myself, but thereafter, when I drove down the Bowery and received the unwelcome and unwanted services, I had no compunction about snarling out the window that if the guy didn't move back, I'd be pleased to relieve him of his foot, and that whether or not he had my number was of little moment to me. I always did look for my erstwhile patient though. I figured I'd feel obliged to give *him* a quarter. But I never did see him again. I suppose that shortly after his discharge, his liver must have disintegrated once and for all.

Then there was Shoeless Joe. I don't recall his real name, but I remember him as Shoeless Joe. He came in sick as hell with Klebsiella pneumonia, a very serious form of lung infection that primarily strikes people who are in some way debilitated. Joe's clothes were in tatters and his shoes were virtually nonexistent. Therefore the nurse tossed the whole mess into the trash can. On such seemingly insignificant decisions and acts are based the mightiest of consequences.

Shoeless Joe proved to be a pretty tough debilitated guy, because within a week he was responding nicely to therapy, and within two weeks, he was well on the way to recovery. He turned out to be an interesting old fellow. He spent a few evenings telling me about his early life as a child and a young man in the Northern Florida panhandle. "Guess that's why I grew up to be a pan-handler," he once chuckled. That warn't no joke, son. If anything could be worse than being a Bowery Bum, it may have been being a Northern Florida panhandler.

Anyway, after a few weeks, Shoeless Joe was cured and ready to go out into the world again. We checked him over, wished him well, and figured we'd be seeing him again soon. How soon we didn't know. When we returned from the clinic in the afternoon, there he was, still in his bed. I asked him what was the matter. "Ain't got no clothes," he said and grinned. "Cain't go out in m' hospital pie-jamas." I clutched my head as I remembered what had happened to his garments, and headed for the phone.

The ward social worker promised quick action, and by the next day she appeared with a full outfit of secondhand duds. Joe put them on and then he tried the shoes. That was the first time I realized how big his feet were. He could squeeze his toes and a little more into the 10's that he had been given.

The social worker made a face as she watched. "Oh, dear," she said. "We don't have any used shoes bigger than these. I'll have to get new ones for him, and that's going to take some time."

I really can't explain exactly what happened next. I tried to understand it even at the time, and couldn't. Apparently, the social service had quick and ready access to secondhand clothing: they obtained it from dead patients or from charitable agencies. However, to get a new, unused article involved the filling out of quintuplicate sets of forms which, for all I know, may have gone as far as the mayor's office. Apparently, they were scrutinized by every welfare superintendent in the five boroughs in order to make absolutely certain that no expense was wasted; that somewhere in New York City there was not a usable secondhand item.

Boy, did they try to save money on Shoeless Joe. He remained in the hospital for five more weeks waiting for his shoes. At first I tried to find out where we stood by calling the social worker. One day the forms were held up in Mr. Bigshot's office. The next day they were being stamped in quintuplicate by Commissioner Broadbeam. After that there was difficulty in locating a pair of shoes enormous enough to fit our patient. No wonder the social workers at Bellevue always looked so haggard. Finally, I just gave up. No one else was unhappy, why should I be?

Shoeless Joe was happy. It was still winter and he had continued access to his warm bed and his three squares a day. The kitchen help was happy, because when the truck was wheeled in with the grub, Shoeless Joe bounded out of bed and served all the customers with a flourish. Then, when they had eaten, he'd collect the trays. The aides and messengers were happy, since Shoeless Joe was only too pleased to help keep the records, or to pick up an item at the Central Supply station. Even the nurses were happy.

Old Shoeless thought nothing of bringing a bedpan to an immobilized comrade and then emptying it and tossing it into the cleaning hopper.

Finally, one morning, the shoes arrived. At least the social worker swore she had left them on the ward. No one else ever saw them. The possibilities are two: either someone swiped them, or Shoeless Joe quietly tossed them into the nearest incinerator. In any case, S.J. remained with us for another week while the social worker hunted up another pair of Gargantua Specials. This time she delivered them personally to Joe and then watched while he put them on. But by now it was March, the sap was a'bustin', and Joe was ready to be on his way. New York City sure did save on him. Hospitalization was not as expensive then as now, so at $40 a day for forty-two days, Joe's shoes cost only $1,680. I must admit, though, they really were nice looking shoes.

One guy who was not really a Bowery Bum deserves to have his story told here. He was a pseudo-bum. He ran afoul of a camel driver, and ended up very dead.

"Camel driver" was a derogatory sobriquet given to some house staff members in some hospitals in and around New York City. By and large, camel drivers were found at smaller, non-university-affiliated hospitals, where they served as cheap labor. They were called camel drivers because frequently they hailed from one of the Arab countries, but this was not invariable, I have also met Chinese and South American camel drivers. To qualify for the title, it was necessary that the doctor (a) show total disregard for human lives and feelings, and (b) have had his training at a school of the caliber of The Deepest Bulgarian Royal Institute of Proctologic Acupuncture. Although it is true that all foreign graduates must pass an examination designed to test their medical qualifications, I strongly suspect that some New York hospitals may have been trafficking in illegal aliens.

My pseudo-bum arrived at Bellevue on one of those very special New York May afternoons. The day before it had been 60°. This day, it was 97° in the shade, and we all were trudging around the hospital with our tongues hanging out, canteens at our waists, and salt pills in our pockets. About two P.M. an ambulance roared up to the door and disgorged an unconscious Negro man, who was promptly zipped into a bed. His referral sheet, from Bronx Puspocket General Hospital had only one word on it: "Psicosis." It was signed by the so-called referring physician. That was the extent of it.

The situation was obvious. One thing that a camel driver is very good at is dumping. This is a practice designed to keep one's workload at minimal levels. You invent some reason why a patient cannot be admitted to your hospital, such as "no beds" or "psychiatric disease" or "communicable disease." Then the patient becomes eligible for transfer to Bellevue, and you go back to sleep and dream happy dreams of oases and date palms.

In this case, I couldn't fathom the reason. Did Dr. Driver mean "psychosis"? Or was this patient known to have been consorting with parrots, and therefore thought to have psittacosis? The question was really unimportant, because what the guy obviously was suffering from was heat stroke. His temperature was 107°. We tried everything we could think of to get it down, but we weren't very successful. Or maybe we were too successful. By that night he was at room temperature, approximately 80°.

I found it upsetting that the lazy or stupid (though the traits are not mutually exclusive) camel driver had sent a man with heat stroke on a forty-five-minute ride in a metal ambulance in 97° weather, a procedure which must have fried the patient's brain for good. I was even more upset when his family finally caught up to his whereabouts. His wife, the kids trailing behind, told me that her husband had been on a construction job in the Bronx, and that when he had fallen sick, the foreman had called for an ambulance to get him quickly to a hospital. It was a good idea, but it was unfortunate that the ambulance had failed to take him to a hospital.

The bummest bum of them all was a fellow I met one Friday night. Since interns worked alternate-night shifts, every other week, we'd work from Thursday morning till Saturday morning, in order to get the weekend off. Therefore, by late Friday night, we'd be more than a bit punchy. It was at this time, and in this state that I went down to the dining room for a midnight snack. There I met my friend Jim Barkley.

Jim was a surgery intern. He was a dour, laconic little fellow whose directness and brusque attitude annoyed many people. I liked him.

Jim was particularly dour and laconic this night, and I asked him what was the matter. He ran his hand through his hair and grimaced. "God damn shithead on my ward's really buggin' me," he mumbled. I asked him to elucidate.

He leaned on his elbow and glowered in my direction. "There's this guy, Mr. Watson," he said. "Biggest pain in the ass you can imagine. Well, he found out the hospital rule that says any time a patient comes in and claims he's been knocked unconscious, you've got to admit him for overnight observation. He's had six admissions in the past two weeks."

"So what, Jim? So you give the guy a bed overnight. What do you care?"

"I'll tell you what I care," he said. "The bastard doesn't just take the bed. Oh, no. He bugs the nurses and pinches their boobs as they go by. Then they wake me up—if I've ever gotten to sleep in the first place—to do something about him. Do something about him! I'd like to kill the son-of-a-bitch."

I was becoming aware of the full gravity of the situation. But Jim wasn't finished. "Not only that," he went on, "but he sneaks over to the other beds and there'll be some poor guy with a new scar on his belly, and he'll tweak him in the scar and then run back to his own bed."

I had an idea. "Jim, why don't you send him to psych?"

"You think I haven't thought of that? Christ, I tried it a long time ago. You know what the Shrink said?"

"No."

"He wouldn't make the transfer. Said Watson wasn't nuts, just mean."

I was feeling sorrier for my poor friend by the minute.

"Well, I finally shipped him out this morning," moaned Jim. "Told him if I ever saw him again, I'd cut his balls off. So he went uptown to Puspocket and gave them the knocked-cold routine."

"Well, how does that affect you?" I asked.

"I'll tell you how it affects me. The camel driver up there shipped him down here a half hour ago. No beds, he said. That's how."

"Jim, we've got to get rid of him." My righteous indignation knew no bounds.

"No way, Larry. He won't leave no matter what I'd do to him." Jim took a long swig of his coffee.

Suddenly I had it. "Listen, Jim. He was knocked cold. So let's work him up."

"What the hell do you mean?"

I began to talk faster. "He says he's been knocked out. Therefore, he needs a spinal tap. Maybe he had a head injury— right?"

"He'll settle for a spinal tap, Larry. He wouldn't give a shit."

"All right, you tell him I'm a new medical student and it's my first case. That'll shake him up."

Jim thought a minute and decided it was worth a try. So we finished our snacks and walked up to his ward.

Jim led me to the bedside of the meanest, nastiest, scowliest, dirtiest bum I'd ever seen. He was just sitting on the edge of his bed, looking professionally malevolent. For a minute I had misgivings. Suppose he took the spinal needle away and killed me with it? I recovered my courage by reminding myself that there were two of us. Jim went through the ritual of introducing me while I shuffled around and looked embarrassed. The guy didn't bat an eye. He signed the permit form for the spinal tap. Then he hawked up an oyster and spat it right on the floor at our feet. If I had needed further selling, I was now sold.

The patient lay calmly as I did my "first" spinal tap. He didn't bat an eye when Jim yelled out such pleasantries as, "My God, don't get that dirt in there; he'll get meningitis." Or, "Stop! Stop! Don't put the needle in so far; you'll paralyze his legs for life." Finally we walked away with our little tube of spinal fluid. The patient favored us with a sneer and sat grinning evilly after us even as we turned the corner.

"I told you it wouldn't work," muttered Jim. "I'm going to grab a few minutes of sleep while I can." He started to leave.

"Wait a minute," I said. "This spinal fluid looks normal, doesn't it?"

"Yeah—so?"

"So we still haven't made sure the knock on the head didn't do him any harm. That means we've got to do a brain biopsy."

Jim looked at me as though I had just flown in the window and announced that I had arrived from Mars. Then he mumbled, "Why the hell not?" He shrugged, and we walked back onto the ward.

The patient glowered at us when we told him our intentions. "What the hell is *that*?" he growled.

"Well, you just take a needle," I said, "and you stick it through the skull up here, where you had your soft spot when you were a baby. Then you take out a little piece of brain in the needle and look to see if it was damaged when you got knocked cold."

"Stick a needle in my head? Shit, don't you come near me, you bastards. I'll kill y' both."

Jim drew himself up full height. "Well, sir," he said. "If you won't allow me to do what needs to be done to check you out after you got knocked cold, I'll have to discharge you."

"I never got none o' these tests before when I got knocked out," growled the patient.

"Well, sir," I said as haughtily as I could, "in that case, you got lousy care."

Jim produced a hospital form for the man to sign which would indicate that he was leaving against medical advice. But he didn't sign. He looked back at us and asked, "How big's the needle—like the one fer the spinal tap?"

"Oh no," I answered. "We need a bigger one than that. It's about this big." I produced my pencil for him to inspect.

He looked at it and shrugged. Then he reached for a pen and began to sign—not the discharge paper, but the permission for the brain biopsy. As he started to write his name, I looked at Jim and he at me.

What were we going to do now? It would have given us both great pleasure to go out and find the biggest trocar we could, and then make a brain-kabob out of the guy, but we felt that we really couldn't do that. For example, how would we dispose of his body? Jim began to walk away in disgust.

"You're very wise, sir," I said. He stopped writing in mid-name and looked at me. "It's not bad at all," I continued. "There's just a brief second of pain and then when the needle goes into your brain, you go like this." I jumped off the ground, flung my arms and legs outward, contorted my face, and screamed, "Blaaaaaaaaa!" at the top of my lungs. "Then you don't feel anything at all."

He stared hard at me. I leered at him. The tide had turned: now it was he who looked scared.

"God damn, I'm gettin' outa here. Gimme that discharge paper."

"Oh no, sir," said Jim. "You signed for the brain biopsy. I want to do it; I've never done one before."

By this time the guy was half dressed. "No sirree, you get the hell away from me. I'm leavin'."

"Well, you know if you sign out against medical advice, you can't ever come back. If you do, you'll have to have the brain biopsy." Thus spake Barkley.

The guy signed the paper and was out the door in a flash. Jim and I shook hands and trundled off to our respective sacks.

Perhaps you find this kind of behavior shocking. Deviance (and deviants) was (and were) tolerated at Bellevue; nonetheless the place was a tenuously balanced society. The filthy surroundings, creaky old equipment, chronic understaffing, and dreadfully sick patients combined to keep us all one step from total chaos. Anyone threatening to needlessly or willfully drop the final straw could not be tolerated. Therefore, occasional individuals had to be evicted. The Bellevue house staffer's genius for eviction frequently bordered on the unbelievable.

This is well illustrated by the story that involved a resident who was one of my friends, a thoroughly humane and kind person. At one time, he and his ward were stuck with one of the relatively rare female bums. She got over her pneumonia, but wouldn't leave the hospital. Whenever discharge seemed imminent, she'd fake a faint or a crushing pain in the chest. This would always be good for another few days in The Vue.

She had no family to take her in. All the city convalescent and nursing homes were full. There was nowhere to send her. Ordinarily, she would have been tolerated as a long-term guest, but she, like Jim Barkley's patient, was a habitual troublemaker. She was prone to midnight screeching when the nurses didn't move fast enough to suit her. She stole food from the other patients and woke them up at night by dropping bedpans on the floor. The sick patients got sicker, and to avoid her the night nurses and aides began to find reasons to spend all their time on other wards. An attempt to transfer her to psychiatry met with the same result: she's not crazy, just impossible.

Faced with the imminent total disintegration of his ward routine and services, the resident felt compelled to act. At four o'clock one morning, he slipped quietly onto the ward, glided over to his tormenter's bed, unzipped his fly, and urinated on her bed sheets. As she let loose the first yodel of protest, he lit out for his room.

Ten minutes later, having been summoned by the nurse, the resident went to the ward and called the psychiatrist again. As the Shrink arrived, the patient pointed a finger at the resident and shrieked, "He peed all over my bed. The doctor peed on my bed!" The resident shrugged and quietly explained that yes, the patient had been incontinent of urine for a while now, but these nocturnal paranoid delusions were relatively new.

The commitment order was signed without further ado, the nasty old woman was carted off, the nurse and aides returned to the ward, and the resident and his patients had their best half-night's sleep in days.

4

The Chicken–Soup–
for–Lunch Bunch

Not only is Bellevue Hospital located close to the Bowery, it is as I've already mentioned, also very near the Lower East Side area of New York. This helps to explain why Jack Thorn, an intern up from Baltimore, said to me one day: "My admissions all seem to have either the Dom or the Lol Syndrome."

"What the hell are those?" I asked him.

"Dom. D.O.M. Dirty Old Man Syndrome. And L.O.L. is Little Old Lady Syndrome."

Jack could justifiably have inserted a J between the O and the second L: Little Old Jewish Lady. This ethnic oddity was explained by the fact that Bellevue was then caring for the last survivors of the once-large Jewish population of the Lower East Side. The increasingly decreasing number of L.O.J.L.'s came to The Vue with their organic and functional *kvetches*, while their children patronized the fency-schmency private hospitals in the fency-schmency Lung Island and New Joisey suboibs to which they had moved. Thus, at Bellevue, for all practical purposes, although every little old lady was not Jewish, every little Jewish lady was old. And their age notwithstanding, more often than not they taxed the ability and understanding of the Bellevue house staff to the very limit.

One of the most inventive L.O.J.L.'s was Mrs. Spray-Me-Dokteh. I first met her about nine o'clock on a September morning during my internship year. We were making rounds with our attending physician, Dr. Carla Slaymaker, when the Emergency Room nurse called to tell us we had an emergency admission. Albert Goodman, the other intern who had also worked on this ward during the previous month, took the call. Immediately upon hanging up, he grabbed an aerosol can of a local anesthetic called Dermoplast. Then he headed for the door. Dr. Slaymaker asked what he needed the Dermoplast for.

"Come on down. I'll show you," he said. So we all came.

When we got to the Emergency Room, Albert led us to the bedside of a short but massive gray-haired lady who was lying profoundly unconscious in her bed. "It's Mrs. Goldberg," he explained. "This is the third time in the last month she's been in with an insulin overdose." As he said this, he drew up a large syringeful of concentrated glucose to inject into her vein.

"But what's the Dermoplast for?" repeated Dr. Slaymaker.

"That's why she takes the insulin overdose," said Albert.

"What?"

"Just watch." He injected the glucose slowly, and within a couple of minutes Mrs. Goldberg's eyes began to flutter open. Before five minutes had passed she was wide awake, and she flashed Albert a broad grin of recognition.

"Dokteh Goodman," she beamed. "DOKteh Goodman! Spray me, Dokteh, spray me."

With that, she lifted her pendulous right breast, releasing a nauseating blast of fetid air. The entire underside of her breast and the subjacent chest wall formed a red, confluent, chronically infected, oozing mess. Albert aimed the Dermoplast at the offending region and let fire. "Ahhh, dot's gud," the patient smiled.

Mrs. Goldberg beamed at Albert, dropped the right breast, and elevated the left one, whose undersurface looked as bad as that of the first one. "Now d'udda one, if you would pliss." Albert promptly anesthetized her left side.

Dr. Slaymaker looked absolutely stricken. "Albert!" she groaned. "You've just got to be kidding."

"No, Dr. Slaymaker. Some time last year, one of the interns kicked her out of the Clinic when she came in for her Dermoplast bottle. Told her if she couldn't dry her breasts and keep them clean, he wouldn't treat her. So now when it bothers her enough, she takes an overdose of insulin to get into the E.R., and then she's got it made."

Mrs. Goldberg confirmed the story by beaming again at Albert and then casting a fierce eye on Dr. Slaymaker. "And Dokteh Goodman's deh nices' dokteh around. He takes gud care uff me!"

Albert beamed back at her and smiled sweetly at Dr. Slaymaker, who shook her head and walked out into the corridor, where she proceeded to laugh until the tears ran.

Another frequent visitor to The Vue was Sadie Abramowitz. Mrs. A. was extremely obese, diabetic, and had high blood pressure and heart disease. She was another lady who was difficult to keep on long-term maintenance therapy. The problem was that when she began to feel well, she would stop taking her digitalis and anti-hypertensive drugs. Then she would promptly go into severe heart failure, whereupon she would be rushed to the hospital. She became known as The Bluebird, because once every month or two, she would appear in the Emergency Room, gasping and cyanotic. But the lady had amazing recuperative powers: a night of emergency measures in the E.R. and she was about as good as new. A couple of days to get her back on her medications and she'd return home. But she never seemed to learn. Not even the time she actually stopped breathing in the corridor leading to the E.R. and had to be cardiac-massaged back to life. A month after this particular episode, she was back again.

Every intern tried every technique he could think of to get her to stay on her pills. Explanations—even in Yiddish—did nothing. No more effective were attempts to embarrass her. We asked her whether she knew the medications were free. She did. One resident called in a psychiatrist to try to determine whether Mrs. A. was nurturing a death wish. After three or four sessions, the Shrink told us that as far as he could tell, her psyche was in order, but that if he continued to see her, he was afraid that he would develop a death wish. All he could tell us was that she just didn't see the need to take medication for her heart when it was doing fine.

A different matter, however, was Mrs. Abramowitz' extremely mild diabetes. She would faithfully test her urine twice a day or more, and would never fail to take her oral medication. Once I asked her the reason for her dichotomous therapeutic philosophy. She gave me the Jewish grandma smile, as though a cookie and milk were coming next, and said, "Dokteh Karp! You know dybeetis kin be dainj'ris." I nodded and then walked around the corner to bang my head against the wall.

One day I tried talking to her husband. Mr. Abramowitz was a skinny little guy with a hatchet face, a hawk's-beak of a nose, a few wisps of scraggly gray hair on top, and a pair of eyes that reflected all the sadness and hostility that can be produced by seventy-two years of absorbing abuse from *goyim*. He always looked like he was swimming in his three-sizes-too-large gray coat with snot on the right sleeve and down the front. He was a pathetic little figure as he ran down the corridors trying to keep up with the stretcher bearers as they raced his wife to the Emergency Room.

"Mr. A.," I said one day, "why doesn't your wife take her heart medicine?"

He gave me a shrug and a go-away notion of his hand.

I tried again. "Don't you know that one of these times we may not be able to get her going again?"

The sadness in his eyes receded and the hostility came forward. "Lissen, sonny, I liff forty-fife yeeihs mit her. *You* vant she should take pills—*you* try liffin mit her. Doan hock me a chinig." (Translation: "Quit bugging me.") I quit bugging him.

I think I won the 1963 Blue Cross Award for the greatest number of admissions of Sadie Abramowitz. She and I eventually got sort of attached to one another. I may have spent more nights with her that year than I did with my wife.

One afternoon during the last week of my internship, as I was sitting on the ward, Mrs. Abramowitz swept in in full sail carrying a gift box, which she proudly unwrapped in front of me. It was a tape recorder, "So you should heff summin to remembeh me mit." I soon saw exactly what she meant; she hooked up the microphone and began to sing into it!

> "Gud bliss Ameh'ika
> Lend det I luff . . ."

A crowd began to gather in the doorway. About fifteen nurses, aides, and patients were watching when Mrs. A., responding to her audience, boomed:

> "Gud bliss Ameh'ika,
> Mein humm, switt humm."

The audience began to applaud, but she waved them into silence. There was more:

> "Gud bliss deh doktehs
> Fer curing mein ill-ness."

I thanked Mrs. Abramowitz as profusely as I could. She left, and I went around the corner to bang my head against the wall again. "Curing mein ill-ness." Jesus Christ!

I didn't realize until several years later that Mrs. A. simply could not accept the fact that her heart was in such bad shape that it needed medication every day for the rest of her life. When she felt well, she stopped the pills, thinking this time maybe it wouldn't come back. Maybe this time they really got rid of it.

Mrs. Gross was an L.O.J.L. who made a very lasting impression in a very short time. She was a scrawny, filthy, incredibly malodorous old lady who was presented to me one Saturday night in the Emergency Room. I walked up to her bed and gagged quietly. Her admitting slip said, "Yetta Gross—? CVA" (that's "possible cerebrovascular accident"—or in plain talk, a stroke). I introduced myself and asked her what had brought her to the hospital.

The little lady looked me square in the eye, inhaled deeply, and let out the most Godawful, piercing shriek I have ever heard:

"MEY-YEH!"

I just stood and stared at her. I guess she thought I needed further explanation, because she then hollered, "MEY-YEH! Y' doity sonuvabitch, y' diditagain! MEY-YEH!"

That's all she said, repeatedly. That was the answer to every question I or anyone else asked her. So we stopped asking her questions. After I had examined her, I got a nurse to help me turn her over to do a spinal tap. As I put the needle in, she let go for what had to be at least the twentieth time: "MEY-YEH! Y' diditagain; y' doity sonuvabitch, y' diditagain. MEY-YEH!" The last syllable lasted fifteen seconds and could have shattered drinking glasses.

A minute later, one of the surgical interns pulled back the curtain around the bed and peered in at Yetta and me. He'd been up all night, his eyeballs looked like a road map of metropolitan New York and I could almost see his nerve ends quivering.

"Karp!" he groaned.

Without looking up from Yetta's dripping spinal fluid, I said, "What?"

"Karp, you listen to me. That screeching is driving me nuts. If you don't shut her up, I'm going to kill her. You understand?" Without waiting for a reply, he snapped the curtain shut and disappeared.

The spinal tap didn't provide the reason for her confused mental state, so I still couldn't tell whether she was sick, senile, or both. As I sat wondering what to do next, she let loose another blast at Meyer. That gave me an idea. I got up and walked out to the waiting room. There sat a guy who could have been Mr. Abramowitz' twin, even to the snot on the shapeless coat. Except for the eyes. They weren't hostile, but rather large, sad, and frightened.

"Is your name Meyer?" I asked.

"Yiz, yiz. Meyeh Guhross."

"Look, I want to ask you about your wife . . . "

"Kin I see her, plizz?" He grabbed me by the lapels, and I thought he was going to cry. I figured, what the hell, he could answer my questions later. Meanwhile, maybe he could shut her up. I led him into the E.R., at which moment Mrs. Gross was once again calling her beloved. We went to her bedside, and Meyer leaned over and patted her head. "I'm here, honey," he murmured.

Yetta turned and gave him a look that turned my blood cold. Her filthy gray hair flew around her white face, and her eyes shot sparks. She sank her nails into his cheeks, and let out with "I'll honey yer ess, y' besstid." With this, Meyer let go a holler, turned tail, and disappeared down the hallway, coattails flying behind him. Yetta sent after him an effort worthy of a goosed Banshee: "MEY-YEH! Y' doity sonuvabitch, y' diditagain. MEY-YEH!" She tried to climb over the bed rails to get her hands on him, and it took two nurses and me to keep the little woman in bed.

At this point the nurses told me that if I didn't have Yetta sent to the psych ward, they'd have me sent. I looked at the two-inch-long, five-track gouge on the hand of one nurse, and called the Shrink. He took one look at and one listen to Mrs. Gross and signed the paper. The orderly wheeled her off strapped into a chair, and we all sank into seats and listened as the echoes and reverberations of "MEY-YEH" became gradually fainter, and finally disappeared forever.

Despite the fact that they were little, the L.O.J.L.'s packed big wallops. One of them was responsible for the most magnificent case of brainwashing I've ever seen: ethnic brainwashing, no less.

She was Mrs. Rosenblatt, an eighty-year-old woman, brought in with (what else?) heart failure. However, she was also suffering from cancer of the vagina, and for this reason she ended up on the gynecology ward. At The Vue, this was a repository for about forty women, many of whom were in varying stages of abortion or suffering from pelvic infections. At least half of them were Puerto Ricans. Amiable and chattery all day, they underwent personality transformations at night. When the lights were shut off, they lay in their beds and realized that they were uncomfortable, lonely, and frightened. Therefore, they'd spend the night softly moaning "Ay!" over and over. When I was called onto the ward at night, it was eerie to walk down the rows of beds while upward of twenty disembodied "Ay's!" converged on me from all directions.

Mrs. Rosenblatt lived for two nights and one day before the combination of the cancer and heart failure did her in. During this time, as she struggled for breath, she uttered only one word: "Oy." Not plaintive like the Puerto Rican Ay, but piercing and demanding, and repeated at about forty-five-second intervals.

During her second night on the ward, while I was giving attention to a Mrs. Gonzales, who was completing her abortion, I realized that the Oys had stopped. I told Mrs. G. I'd be right back, and went over to find the reason for the silence. The reason being apparent, I went right back to Mrs. Gonzales.

After she had finished miscarrying, I returned to the front of the ward to get the name and number of Mrs. Rosenblatt's next of kin. At that point it suddenly occurred to me that something was wrong. I stopped and listened. From every corner of the room came soft, plaintive Oys. Not Ays. Oys. By the next night though, all was back to normal, and Spanish again replaced Yiddish as the official language of the Bellevue gynecology ward. *Sic transit gloria! Sic semper tyrannis!*

My most memorable L.O.J.L. was Zelda Katzman. Mrs. Katzman was sixty-eight years old. Her frontal balding, small thick neck, huge bulging eyeballs, and pot belly combined to give her the appearance of a gigantic frog. This was reinforced by her grating, guttural voice. Her hair—natural gray interspersed with dyed orange-red—simply added a grotesque fillip to her presence.

Mrs. Katzman was a frequent visitor to our wards. She invariably came in complaining of chest pain and shortness of breath. Physical examination, X-rays, and cardiograms were always normal, with the exception of some minor findings consistent with bronchitis and emphysema. So she'd be kept in the hospital for three to ten days for observation and tests. The observations were monotonously normal and so were the tests. No heart disease was ever found. Because of her obesity, dry skin, hair loss, and constipation (the latter a symptom without which one could not be properly labeled an L.O.J.L.), every new set of interns worked her up for hypothyroidism. This workup also was invariably normal. She must have been the only lady in the history of The Vue or any other place with twenty negative workups for thyroid disease.

Mrs. Katzman had one especially annoying quality. As are most patients with emphysema, she was a chronic smoker. Therefore, on admission, her cigarettes were always confiscated. That meant war.

During the day, Zelda made her mooching rounds, managing to collect five or ten cigarettes from the other patients. Then she'd stash them away. We never could find her hiding place. But when the midnight-to-eight shift rolled around, Zelda would creep past the dozing aides, go into the bathroom, and make like a furnace.

From that point on, the sequence was absolutely predictable and totally repeatable. About a half hour after going in, she'd stagger out of the bathroom with her nicotine nerves pacified, but wheezing and gasping for breath. She'd make it as far as the nursing station, and there collapse to her knees. With what would sound like a terminal effort, she'd lift her pop eyes to the nurse or the aide and announce in her Andy Devine baritone:

"Call d'dokteh! I'm gunna *faint!*"

This call usually would awaken the intern after about an hour's sleep. He'd stagger crankily down to the ward and revive Zelda with a few whiffs of oxygen and a dose of phenobarb. Then, lifting her protuberant eyes in deepest gratitude, she'd offer thanks and homage to her savior physician and promise never, never to touch the vile weed again. Which vow she would keep for the remainder of the night. You could say that much for Zelda: she never woke up a dokteh more than once a night. Undoubtedly because she'd run out of cigarettes on the first go-round.

We tried every available technique to break Mrs. Katzman of her habit: persuasion, argument, threats, tearful pleas, but all had the same effect. Zelda would fill her frog eyes with all the innocence she could muster, avow total agreement, and promise obedience from then on. Then we'd go off on our rounds and she'd go off on hers. We were grateful that her stays on the ward, though frequent, were brief.

The last time I saw Zelda she was gasping in the emergency

room while another intern, who had not yet met her, was frantically pushing oxygen into her with one hand and taking an electrocardiogram with the other. When Zelda saw me walk by, she waved and yelled, "Yoo-hoo. Dokteh Kahp!" I grinned at her and went over. "I'm beck," she said. "I vuz heffen trubble mit breeding again."

"I see, Mrs. Katzman." Then I added, "I'll tell your new doctor about you, so he'll know your case."

"Ah . . . dot vould be nice."

Her new doctor had stopped in mid-cardiogram, and stood staring at her in utter disbelief, the cardiogram paper continuing to roll out and onto the floor. I told him that Mrs. Katzman was a frequent visitor to his new ward, that she had severe episodes of shortness of breath that came and went without apparent cause or explanation, that no one yet had been able to find any disease other than her emphysema, and that she smoked too much. . . .

"Now, Dokteh Kahp (the forefinger waved a la Molly Goldberg), you dunt heff to tell him effryt'ing," she interrupted.

. . . and that for a few days he would have to make sure there was nothing new, and then he could, with clear conscience, discharge her. I also told him that he could save a lot of his time and even more of her blood by forgetting about her thyroid gland. Then I bid Mrs. K. good-bye.

A few days later I was eating lunch when this same doctor came up to me and asked me whether I remembered Mrs. K. I assured him I did.

"Well," he said, "I worked her up and couldn't find a thing wrong with her, except for the emphysema, like you said. But she drove us all crazy with this damn habit she had of sneaking smokes at night . . . "

"What do you mean had?" I asked. "She'll have that habit till she dies."

"She *is* dead," he said.

"She's *what?*"

"I sent her out this morning, all chipper and cheerful. She got as far as the front steps, Larry, and she just keeled over. She was D.O.A. when they brought her back in."

I pushed my plate away and just sat for a whole minute without moving. Finally I muttered, "Well, that's one autopsy I'm going to watch. I've got to know what the hell she had."

"No autopsy, Larry."

"Why not?"

"Family wouldn't allow it. One of the daughters grabbed me by the tie and began to scream that first we had killed her mother and now we wanted to cut her open and make her suffer more."

I angrily left the table and went up to my room to kick my wastebasket. Then I went back to work. The next day they buried Zelda with her secret, and all I could do was gnash my teeth.

So it went, on and on, seemingly without end. Fourteen years ago the L.O.J.L.'s were a basic part of patientry at The Vue. However, attrition and medical insurance plans will soon take their full toll, and the Bellevue L.O.J.L. will have to be declared an endangered species. In not too many years, an intern may actually have to walk down the street to Beth Israel Hospital, just to see one. Evolution is a harsh process, and its inevitability cannot be denied.

5

Gays, Too, Came to The Vue

In recent years, homosexuals and homosexuality have begun to come out into the open. Although many people still clear their throats uncomfortably when the subject arises, the increasing candor may be starting to diminish the persecution that homosexuals have long suffered.

In the early 1960's, however, gay had not yet become beautiful. As a matter of fact, homosexuals hadn't even become gays. They were still called queers and fairies, and in the Bellevue neighborhood, one usually heard them referred to as doity fags. It was considered great sport among the local bucks to beat them to bloody pulps, and then take their money and valuables.

Homosexuals have always had special medical problems, but the prejudice against them frequently militated against their obtaining care. They knew that they were not welcome in most private doctors's offices: it would have given the places a bad name. Hence, as was the case with the alcoholics, the bums, the prostitutes, and the penniless, Bellevue became the homosexuals' last resort. No one was ever turned away at The Vue, and most of the young house-staff members could be counted on to be considerably less judgmental than older members of the medical fraternity.

Thus, homosexuals were seen frequently in the Bellevue Admitting Office and on the wards, and we came to look upon them with a reasonably casual attitude. When you came right down to it, their habits were no more peculiar than those of the great majority of our patients.

My first encounter with a homosexual and his particularly homosexual problem occurred while I was serving my internship rotation in the Admitting Office. About two o'clock one morning, the nurse handed me a treatment slip on which she had written "FB." This was the abbreviation for "foreign body," and when written in such a non-specific manner it usually meant that the complainant had a cinder in his eye. I couldn't figure out why the nurse was smirking as she handed me the slip.

I walked into the examining room, where I found a young man in his twenties. He was wearing a tight-fitting pair of chinos and a suede jacket over a white T-shirt. His hair was blond and curly, considerably longer than what was fashionable in 1963. His hands were clenched in his lap, his lips were tightly drawn.

"Got a little something in your eye?" I asked.

At that, his face broke up and he started to chortle. His amusement seemed odd and inappropriate to my question, and I involuntarily stepped back a pace. My expression must have transmitted my dismay, because the patient made an effeminate "never mind" gesture with his hand and said, "Please don't take offense, Doctor. It just sounded like they hadn't taught you your anatomy very well. You *were* joking, of course, weren't you?"

I took a quick look at the treatment slip; it certainly did say "FB." But then the vagueness of the terminology struck me, especially since it was more than apparent what this fellow's sexual preferences were.

"I . . . I'm sorry," I said slowly, holding up the treatment slip for reference. "All this paper says is that your problem is some sort of foreign object, but it doesn't say where. I assumed it was in your eye."

The man broke into laughter again. "Oh, *Doctor*," he said. I'm afraid your nurse was being, shall we say, a little delicate? Actually, to be quite blunt about it, my problem is that I've got a Coke bottle stuck up my ass."

I fought fiercely to keep a straight face, but the battle was lost before it had even begun. My patient, both satisfied that I was not angry, and pleased to have brightened my nocturnal hours, said, "Shall I tell you how it got there?" He smirked, looking very much like the nurse had looked when she handed me the treatment slip.

"No, that won't be necessary," I answered. Although I had never before personally encountered such a situation, the Bellevue scuttlebutt had been sufficient in educating me. Homosexuals engage in anal intercourse, and as the sphincter of the anus becomes stretched by repeated dilation, the sex act becomes less and less satisfactory. Therefore, prostheses of greater dimensions are used. Greased bananas are reportedly a favorite, but after a while they too become less than satisfying. At that point, soda bottles come into use, and with their gradually increasing diameters, it becomes sort of a measure of gay macho to see how much of the bottle the recipient can tolerate. Apparently I was dealing with a highly talented individual but, unfortunately, his partner must have developed slippery fingers at a highly inopportune moment.

I told my patient to disrobe for examination. Then I put on a glove and smeared some lubricating jelly over my index finger. In a rectal examination, the anal sphincter usually permits the examining finger to pass only with considerable reluctance, to say nothing of discomfort on the part of the patient. In this case, though, there was no resistance or discomfort whatever. I probably could have put all five fingers through, but there was nowhere for them to go. Directly inside the anal opening was the bottle.

I cursed as I felt its surface and realized that the bottom was facing me; I had been hoping that the bottle just might have been inserted base first so that I would be able to hook a finger inside the neck and pull it out. For approximately fifteen minutes I tried to extract the bottle by inserting both index fingers, one on each side, and pulling outward. All I accomplished, though, was to make the bottle spin around within the rectum.

Finally I decided it was time to call in the reserves, so I took off my gloves, walked across the hall, and told my story to Henry Kaufman, the surgical resident. Henry grinned. "Your first Coke Bottle, huh?" he said. "Well, it won't be your last, you work around here long enough. Come on, I'll show you how to do it. These guys got assholes like you can't believe: they really stretch out. You can't be afraid to pull a little: just pull straight out, not sideways, and you'll never rupture a rectum."

We walked back into my patient's room, Henry put on gloves, and then he went to work. Slowly, gingerly, he slid in the middle three fingers of each hand. Then he braced himself and began to pull. The bottle bulged against the attenuated sphincter, and as it did, Henry's hands came together in the midline with an audible slap. The bottle squirted upward, and the patient let out a yelp.

Henry stepped back, almost scratched his head, but recovered himself just in time, "Hmm," he mused. "Bend over and let's try again." Henry tried again, but the result was the same.

"This is the god-damndest slipperiest bottle I've ever seen," Henry said to me, a puzzled look on his face.

Suddenly I realized why. All that lubricating jelly I had used on my fingers had been transferred to the bottle, making it as slippery as the proverbial greased pig. My feeling of chagrin was not lessened when the patient slipped me a sly wink.

"I'll be right back," Henry said. "I'm going up to OB for a minute."

"OB?" I asked. I couldn't imagine why Henry would be going to the obstetrics floor at that point.

"Just don't go away," he said, as he walked briskly out the door.

A few minutes later Henry returned carrying a contraption I have since become thoroughly familiar with, but which at the time was utterly foreign to me. "This is called a vacuum extractor," he said, as he walked in. "It's used sort of like forceps, to pull a baby out. This little cup here fits on the top of the baby's head, and the vacuum pump, over here, creates a suction through the hose. Then you just pull on the hose, and out comes the baby. Or in this case, the Coke bottle."

"Jesus God," I said. "Did you tell the OB resident what you were going to use his baby-schlepper for?"

"As a matter of fact, I did," said Henry. "I know the guy who's on tonight pretty well, and he's kind of a character. He thought it was a pretty clever idea. Actually he wanted to come down to watch, except he had a lady all ready to deliver."

Henry checked the assembly of the vacuum extractor, and then set about trying to apply the metal cup to the base of the Coke bottle. But every time he pushed the cup against the bottle, the latter would float deeper into the rectum, and he was never able to achieve a tight enough seal to permit him to pump up the vacuum. Finally, his face bright red and dripping sweat, he put down the instrument and shook his head sadly.

"Do you think we could get a pair of obstetric forceps and use them to pull it out?" I asked hopefully.

Henry shook his head again. "They're too big," he said. "I'm afraid we might put the end of one right through the rectum." His face brightened. "But maybe we could get a high-speed drill from maintenance, make a hole in the bottom, and hook a stick or something through it."

"That doesn't sound wise," I said. "For one thing, the glass slivers up there might not do him too much good. And for another, if the bottle wouldn't hold still for the vacuum cup, it's not very likely to hold still for the drill bit."

"I wish you guys would figure *something* out," said the patient, a little querulously. "I know it's my own fault, but I really don't want to go through the rest of my life with this bottle up my ass."

Henry jumped up and slapped the man on the shoulder. "Don't worry, old fellow," he said. "We're going to get your bottle out for you all right. But we'll have to put you to sleep to do it." Then he turned to me. "Arrange for anesthesia and an operating room," he said, "and call me when they're ready to put him to sleep."

A couple of hours passed before I could take care of all the preliminaries which are necessary before someone can receive general anesthesia, but finally we were all set, and I gave Henry a call. After the patient was rendered unconscious, we strapped him to the operating table in the prone position, with his knees drawn up against his chest. Then the anesthetist, at Henry's order, lowered the foot of the table so that gravity would be of maximal help in the procedure.

With a bit of a flourish, Henry produced a pair of rubber gloves, two squares of yellow sponge rubber, a roll of cellophane tape, and a pair of bandage scissors. While I watched, entranced, he put on the gloves and then proceeded to cut out finger-sized pieces of the sponge rubber, which he taped to his gloved digits. This done, he inserted the middle three fingers of each hand into the patient's anus, as he had previously done in the A.O. Squeezing the Coke bottle so tightly that his teeth were clenched, he pulled. This time, with the improved traction provided by the sponge rubber, the bottle slowly emerged through the sphincter. Henry held it aloft in triumph.

The anesthetist whistled appreciatively. "Twelve full ounces, that's a lot," he said.

The Great Coke Bottle Extraction was a sweaty affair for a while, but it was a minor venture compared to the matter of Arthur Arisburi's rectal miseries. Arthur was a slight young man with sandy hair that hung forward into his eyes, and when he staggered into the Admitting Office, he appeared to be about a step and a half in front of the old fellow with the scythe. He made it to the nurse's desk, moaned, "My stomach . . . " and collapsed in front of her. She motioned to a guard who was standing in the corner. The guard hurried over, picked Arthur up under the arms, and dragged him into an examining room. Meanwhile, the nurse rushed into the room where I was culturing up a strep throat to tell me my talents were needed elsewhere, *prontissimo*.

An aide was undressing Arthur as I walked in. I stood and watched as they slipped a gown onto him. He lay on his side, legs drawn up to his chest, clutching his belly, and rocking gently back and forth. I put my hand on his shoulder to draw his attention, and asked him what was the matter.

His eyes were glassy as he looked up at me. "My stomach . . . hurts real bad," he whispered. The very effort of saying the words seemed to cause him pain.

"When did it start?" I asked.

"Few . . . hours . . . ago," he answered.

"Have you had any nausea. Vomiting?"

Gingerly, he shook his head yes.

I told him to turn over onto his back so I might examine his abdomen. He winced.

"I'm sorry," I said. "But that's the only way I can try to find out what's wrong."

It hurt me to watch him roll over, but finally he made it, lying on his back, breathing shallowly and rapidly, with knees pointing toward the ceiling. When I placed my hand to the right of his navel, he screamed in agony and then shivered violently.

I was puzzled. This man had all the signs of acute peritonitis, but had a normal blood pressure and temperature. That ruled against an infectious cause for his problem, and I wondered whether he was suffering from a perforated peptic ulcer, with spillage of stomach acid into the peritoneal cavity. Such a catastrophe would also have permitted the entry of free air into the peritoneal cavity through the hole in the stomach, so I had Arthur wheeled over to the X-ray department for films. When he returned, I slid the pictures up onto the view box. I had been right on the ball! Under each diaphragm was a clearly delineated pocket of air.

Clutching my roentgenologic triumph, I went into the hallway and collared Randy Braxton, the surgery resident on A.O. call that evening. "What do you think of this?" I said smugly, as I held the X-rays up to a nearby gooseneck lamp.

Randy pursed his lips as he stared at the films. "Has he got the clinical signs of a perforated viscus?" he asked.

"He sure as hell does," I answered. "I figure it must be an ulcer. Come on in; I'll let you look him over for yourself."

When Randy and I walked into the room where they were keeping Arthur under observation, the nurse stage-whispered: "Dr. Karp." As we turned in her direction, she pointed at the stretcher that Arthur had been lying on to go to and from X-ray. Right in the middle was a little puddle of blood.

Randy walked quickly over to Arthur and told him to roll off his back and onto his side again. Slowly, Arthur complied. Randy bent over and peered from below as he spread the patient's buttocks. I watched intently from behind. The entire area around the anus was bloodstained.

"Gimme a glove and some jelly," Randy called to the nurse. "Let's do a rectal and see where this blood's coming from."

Arthur moaned like a poleaxed cow. "No, no," he pleaded. "Don't examine me there. Please."

"You're bleeding from there," Randy said coolly. "I just want to put my finger inside. That may show us what's going on with you."

"No, please don't," whined Arthur. "It just hurts too much there."

Suddenly the vision of a giant Coke bottle materialized in my mind.

"Listen, Arthur," I said, "maybe this sounds a little silly, but you didn't put anything up there, did you?" Arthur remained very quiet. Randy craned his neck at the X-rays, looking for a foreign object in the region of the rectum.

"Come on," I said. "Why don't you tell us what you did. If you don't know it, you're a pretty sick guy, and you may save your life. At least you may save yourself a rectal examination."

Arthur looked up at me, his eyes full of fear. "You wouldn't kick me out of here, would you?" he whimpered.

"Christ, no one ever gets kicked out of Bellevue," I said. "Don't you know that?"

Randy put on his examining glove with a snap.

"All right, all right," cried Arthur. "I'll tell you. A few of us were fooling around a little, you know, at a Gulf station up First Avenue a-ways. We were taking turns sticking the air hose up each other's ass and blowing in a little air. It feels kinda funny, you know? Anyway, one of the guys decided to get wise; I didn't know it. He turned the meter all the way up before he gave me my kick." The little man winced in recollection. "Oh, I tell you, Doctor, I never felt such terrible pain in all my life. I thought he had blown me up."

In fact, that was precisely what Arthur's friend had done. They had been playing a game that some people called homosexual roulette: blowing air into their rectums from a gas-station hose. It was not an uncommon practice, and as one might imagine, injuries were not infrequent. But Arthur's was in a class by itself.

Randy's surgical team operated on him without delay, and found his rectum literally in shreds. He had peritonitis because the blast of air had sent a fecal aerosol spraying throughout his abdominal cavity. It was touch and go for several days, but Arthur finally survived, though with his rectum resected, he was left with a colostomy as a souvenir. An impacted Coke bottle would have been a bargain.

Generally speaking, homosexuals seemed to have trouble with their orifices. If it wasn't the anus, it was the mouth. This latter situation was illustrated by one of our admissions during my tenure as intern on male medicine. He was a tall, very asthenic Chinese man who minced and pranced around the ward, causing the nurses and aides to collapse in helpless laughter. One of them teasingly offered to chaperone me while I examined him.

The patient's name was Charlie Wong, and his problem was a high fever and a sore throat. That didn't sound like anything special, and I wondered why the doctor in the Admitting Office had seen fit to admit him. As I examined him, however, I stopped wondering. Aside from his 104° temperature, he had a chain of swollen lymph glands the size of walnuts running the length of his neck on the left. And his sore throat looked like no strep infection I had ever seen. The entire left tonsilar region was covered with a very angry-looking red sore which was sending out rays of beefy inflammation so that the whole thing looked like a sunburst. Beneath the sore, the throat was so swollen it appeared ready to pop.

Charlie told me that he had been feeling increasingly ill for about a week, with progressive soreness and inability to swallow, and increasing malaise. I couldn't begin to imagine what manner of dread disease he had. I swabbed his lesion, made smears, and examined them under the microscope, but I was unable to identify any particular offending bacterium. I thought that the swelling might be an abscess, but after a good deal of poking around, during which time I had poor Charlie swinging from the chandeliers, I was convinced it was merely a severe tissue reaction to the overlying sore, and not a pus pocket. I wondered whether Charlie might have been suffering from leukemia: such patients are subject to unusual types of infection, often of a fungal origin. However, his blood count was characteristic only of infection, and so, with relief, I scratched blood cancer from my list of diagnostic possibilities. Once again I swabbed the sore and prepared cultures for every microorganism I could think of. Then I called my resident, Arnie Handelman, to take a look.

Arnie made a face as he peered down Charlie's throat. "God, I don't know," he muttered. "I've never seen a lesion like that before."

"That makes two of us," I said.

"It really is an ugly thing, isn't it?" said Arnie. "I'd sure as hell hate to have something like that in *my* throat." He paused a moment. "Which makes me think," he continued slowly, "maybe it could be contagious?"

All of a sudden my entire body began to itch fiercely. I scratched at my left shoulder.

"Let's get a dermatology consultant," said Arnie.

"Now?" I asked. "At ten o'clock at night? What dermatologist is going to come see a patient at this hour?"

"He won't like it," said Arnie. "But he'll come. He has to, since we want him to check out a possible communicable disease. Go ahead and call him."

The dermatology resident was indeed cranky about the after-hours consultation, but he did come and look at Charlie's throat. He, too, grimaced as he inspected the sore, and then he shook his head. "Beats hell out of me," he said. "Did you do a Gram stain?"

"Sure," I answered. "But it didn't show anything."

Our pimple-popping friend shook his head again. "I just don't know," he said. "But it really doesn't look like anything that would be contagious by an airborne route. Why don't you just isolate him in a corner bed with a screen around him and observe handwashing precautions. Then wait for your cultures to come back and see what you get."

"You think we ought to start him off on a broad-spectrum antibiotic in the meanwhile?" Arnie asked.

"I wouldn't," said the dermatologist. "He's got a fever, but he doesn't look at all toxic. Better wait a day or two to check the cultures; if you end up having to culture him up any more, you may get inaccurate results if he's on antibiotics."

So we sent Charlie to the farthest reaches of the ward, put a screen around his bed, and ordered his temperature to be taken every four hours. I went back to the intern's quarters and scrubbed myself in the shower until my skin was raw.

For the next day and a half, Charlie Wong's temperature fluctuated between 98° and 103°, but he continued to feel well, except for his local symptoms. On the afternoon of his second day on our ward, the reports on his throat cultures came back. They were all negative. During rounds that afternoon, Charlie received only the most perfunctory of greetings. Not only was he making us feel unpleasantly incompetent, but the more negative findings that accumulated, the more mysterious his ailment became, and the less anyone wanted to get close to him.

After we had finished rounds, Arnie and I were sitting in the ward examining room entering notes on charts. Suddenly Arnie stopped, put his pen in his mouth, and looked thoughtful. "I've got an idea," he said.

"About Charlie Wong?"

"Yeah. You know what I'm going to do? I'm going to call Dr. Erickson over to take a look at him."

Naturally I wondered why I hadn't thought of that. Dr. Erickson was the dean of the dermatology staff at The Vue, a stocky little man, not much taller than five feet, with a bald head full of wisdom, and with blue eyes from which emanated considerably more mischief than one would expect in a seventy-year-old. When Arnie got him on the phone, he said he'd be glad to come by first thing in the morning.

We were all waiting for him when he strode onto the ward at eight o'clock. Arnie described The Mysterious Case of Charlie Wong, and when he had finished, Dr. Erickson asked one question:

"This patient, is he what you fellows might call ... a little bit on the faggoty side?"

A couple of snickers in our rank answered the question, but I said, anyway, "We're quite certain he is."

"What made you ask that?" said Arnie.

"Let's just go see the patient," replied Dr. Erickson.

As we walked to the back of the ward, Dr. Erickson kept up a nonstop banter, making fun of us for being so afraid of a homosexual that we had to hide him behind a curtain at the rear of the ward. He told us he wanted to make certain that we knew that homosexuality was not catching.

Arnie introduced Dr. Erickson to Charlie, and the old man took out a tongue blade and a flashlight and peered into the patient's throat. As he did, a truly wicked smile broke out on his face.

"Aha, young man!" he fairly bellowed. "I know what *you've* been doing."

Charlie turned bright red and grinned sheepishly. The members of the house staff looked around at each other. One pair of shoulders after another shrugged.

Dr. Erickson patted Charlie on the shoulder, assured him that he'd soon be feeling better and then led us back to the front of the ward. There he explained that Charlie's sore was a very typical chancre, a primary syphilitic lesion. "Every one of you would have recognized it if it had been on his genitals," he said. "But you never stopped to think that homosexuals engage in, shall we say, sexual acts that are a little different. Therefore, they can get chancres in the rectum, or in the mouth and throat. Gentlemen, you must learn to keep your minds open."

Dr. Erickson was right on target. Charlie's bacterial cultures had been negative because the organism which causes syphilis is very fragile outside the human body, and difficult to grow. But when we went back, scraped the lesion, and examined the scrapings under a dark-field microscope, we found battalions of the characteristic corkscrew-shaped bugs. After that, a little penicillin, and Charlie was as good as new.

Very different was the case of Sylvia Pancoast. Sylvia was in her early fifties, and even her dyed hair and about a pound of facial makeup couldn't disguise the fact that she had a foot and a half in the grave. Her eyes were sunken and lusterless, the skin was drawn tightly over her cheekbones, and every detail of every bone in her body stood out in relief under her skin. Her general build suggested that she had once been a strong, even muscular, woman, but that had been before her lung cancer had gone to work on her. The cancer was obvious on her X-rays, and it was also clear that the lesion was beyond all help. She sat patiently as I examined her, wheezing with each breath, but when it came time to do the pelvic exam, she demurred with a vigor that amazed me. "No man ain't gonna put anything in there on me," she said firmly.

I considered the situation for a moment. "Would you like me to call a lady doctor?" I asked. "Would that make you feel better?"

"No sir; no sir!" said Sylvia. "You ain't gonna call no doctor, man or lady. I never did let no one ever touch me down there, and I ain't about to start now."

Once again, I considered. It didn't seem reasonable to pursue the issue: with what Sylvia had growing in her chest, it didn't really matter much what she had in her pelvis. I couldn't see any purpose in trying to force or persuade a dying woman to submit to a pelvic examination. So I omitted the pelvic from my writeup, and when I presented the case to the resident, I also skipped the pelvic part. I figured that Sylvia was either an extremely stalwart virgin or an old butch who just wanted to give me a tough time.

During the subsequent week and a half that Sylvia lived on the ward, we simply tried to keep her comfortable with narcotics. Every morning we said hello to her, and reordered her medications. The last thing on my mind or anyone else's was her unfathomed pelvis.

Finally the evening came when the nurse called to inform me that Sylvia had stopped breathing. I went down to the ward and officially certified that fact. Then I went to the chart rack to make the final entry into Sylvia's folder, and to see whether there were any next of kin to be called. Meanwhile, the nurse and the aide began to prepare the body to be shipped down to the morgue.

I was in the middle of writing my note when I was interrupted by a shriek in the purest hi-fi stereophonic sound. I dropped the chart and started running. The nurse and the aide met me halfway. Each seemed to be trying to outdo the other in generating hysteria; they were screaming and gesticulating wildly. Finally the aide managed to direct my attention to Sylvia's bed, as she yodeled, "Dr. Karp! Oh, Dr. Karp! She's a he—a man!"

I galloped over to Sylvia's body. The reason for her reluctance to have a pelvic examination was plainly evident. She very obviously had been a man, and one with a real problem. She had been a transsexual, an individual who believes he has been trapped or imprisoned within the body of a member of the opposite sex. Sylvia probably took estrogens to feminize her physical characteristics, and she may have undergone electrolysis to remove most of her facial and body hair. It certainly was a good job; it had all of us thoroughly fooled.

Today Sylvia might have been eligible for a sex-change

operation so that she'd have been able to live entirely as a woman. In 1963, though, such procedures were extremely difficult to come by, and the vast majority of transsexuals were forced to practice the kinds of deception that in the end permitted Sylvia to die among the women of Bellevue Hospital rather tha among the men.

Homosexuals and their difficulties turned up in some unlikely parts of The Vue. For example, there was the case of Charlene McGinnis. Charlene was one of my obstetrics patients.

She was a dainty little woman who couldn't have weighed more than a hundred pounds, but when I first saw her on the labor and delivery suite, she was letting out noises worthy of a bull moose in rut. Charlene had been wheeled up from the Admitting Office, where she had presented herself with a severe stomachache, nausea, and vomiting. It had been determined without undue difficulty that these symptoms were those of labor, and she was therefore shipped in haste to us. The intensity of Charlene's howls alarmed me, and I examined here immediately; the exam revealed that the baby was ready to be born. As we proceeded toward a delivery room, I asked, "Is this your first baby."

Charlene stopped roaring long enough to look at me in wonder, and say breathlessly, "are you telling me I'm going to have a baby?"

I thought she was kidding. "What do you think you're carrying around in here," I asked, patting her on the belly, "a basketball?"

"Some of my friends have been telling me I was putting on weight," she answered. "In fact, I had myself on a diet a few weeks ago, but I haven't been able to lose a pound. Actually, I gained three last week alone." At that point, she started to cry.

I administered a saddle block anesthetic, which relieved her of her pains, but the tears kept coming. I though I understood the situation. "What's the matter?" I asked. "You don't have a husband?"

She shook her head. "I never even dreamed I could be pregnant," she said, wiping her forearm across her eyes. "I never felt any movement, and I wasn't sick a day, at least till this afternoon. Now what in the world am I going to do with a baby?"

As I talked, I was getting ready to perform the delivery. "Seems like you've got two choices," I said, as I pulled on my gloves. "You can either keep it or you can have it adopted out. I admit it's a hell of a time to start making that sort of decision, but I don't see how it can be helped. Anyway, you'll have a few days to decide after you deliver. Which reminds me: Do you think you'll want to see the baby, or would you want to do some thinking first?"

"Oh, no," Charlene said rapidly. "I want to see it. I don't think I'll believe I had it unless you show it to me."

Charlene's situation was not as unusual as I thought at the time; I've since been involved in three or four similar cases. At the root of the problem is the psychological mechanism of denial. A young, unmarried girl, to whom pregnancy would be a thorough disaster, subconsciously refuses to accept the possibility that she might in fact be in a family way. She suppresses recognition of all the usual symptoms of pregnancy and carries on, merely believing that she's gaining a bit too much weight. This self-deception continues until the inevitable labor ensues, at which time the true state of affairs can no longer be denied.

I delivered Charlene, uneventfully, of a normal seven-pound boy. She surprised me by showing considerable affection for her new offspring, even to the point of cooing at great length. To put it mildly, her behavior would have caused much pain to those who deny the existence of maternal instincts.

After I had sewed up Charlene's bottom, the nurse wheeled the baby to the nursery. As I was taking off my gown and gloves, my patient called out, "Oh—Dr. Karp."

I asked her what was on her mind.

"I was just wondering," she said. "My friend is outside; she came to the hospital with me. Would you tell her about my baby for me?"

"Better than that," I answered, "let's get you on this stretcher here, and I'll wheel you out to the ward. You can tell her yourself, on the way."

In retrospect, I recalled that Charlene looked a little dubious at that point. But she said okay.

As we went through the swinging doors into the corridor between labor and delivery and the ward, a woman stepped forward from against the wall. Her girth rivaled her height. She had close-cropped, mouse-colored hair, and she was wearing no makeup. Furthermore, it did not take an unusual degree of perception to see that she was smoking mad.

Charlene said, "Hi, Paula," but got no further. Paula waddled up to the side of the stretcher, bellowed, "You've been unfaithful to me!" and delivered Charlene a slap across the cheek that caused the entire stretcher to vibrate.

For a moment I stood there in fascination, watching the drama unfold. Paula proceeded to grab Charlene by the ear, and pummeled her about the head while yelling at the top of her lungs that she was going to teach a good lesson to her unfaithful little bitch. At that point I decided that intervention was necessary, so I grabbed Paula around the midsection and managed to wrestle her off her friend. By now, both women were in tears and near hysteria.

"Get out of here," I said to Paula, pointing at the stairs. "Go on home until you get yourself under control. Then you can come back."

"Huh!" she snorted. "You can't kick me outa here."

"Maybe not," I said, "but the guards can, and they will, if I tell them you were beating up on one of the patients." Once again, I pointed to the stairs.

Paula snorted again. "I'll be back later, dear," she said sarcastically. At first I thought that she was talking to me, but then I realized she was looking directly at Charlene.

She did come back later, and she had indeed cooled off. So much so that she showered Charlene with kisses and told her she had decided to forgive her. Charlene, for her part, accepted her friend's apology and spent the rest of the evening on the ward in her arms, cooing at her in the same tone of voice she had used earlier on her baby.

The next morning, on rounds, Charlene proudly told me that she had made her decision. "We're going to keep the baby and bring him up," she said.

"We?" I asked, knowing too well the answer.

"Oh, yes. Paula just loved the baby when she saw him. She said she thought it'd be nice to have a baby in the house. And she says we can bring him up as well as any *man* and woman could."

"Well," I said, and stopped there, except for a bit of hemming and hawing. "Oh, hell," I finally burst out. "Look, Charlene, do you, uh, really think that's a good idea?"

She looked at me, all innocence.

"I mean, with you and Paula being . . . well, the way you are, do you really think you can do a good job of raising a little boy?"

Charlene looked as though *I* had slapped her. "Paula told me you doctors wouldn't approve of it," she wailed. "But I thought maybe *you* were different." She rolled over in bed to face the wall and started to cry.

"I'm sorry, Charlene," I said. "But think it over a little, would you, please?"

During the next couple of days, whether or not Charlene thought about it, her mind didn't seem to do any changing. She and Paula fussed over the baby, took turns giving him his bottle, and argued over who was going to get to change the next diaper. Finally, I went down to speak to the social worker; I outlined the case to her, and she promised to look into it.

She came back to see me the same afternoon, shaking her head sadly. "I don't think there's anything we can do, Dr. Karp," she said. "It's awfully hard to take a baby away from its natural mother; you have to prove she's totally unfit. And all we've got is an unmarried mother and a woman who claims to be nothing more than her good friend who's going to take her in, shelter her, and help her care for her new baby. That story could melt the heart of any judge in New York City."

"They're a bit more than good friends," I said.

"You may know that," replied the social worker, "but you can't prove it. No one else witnessd their little lovers' quarrel after the baby was born. And they haven't done anything on the ward that they couldn't justify as just affection between two good friends. Furthermore, there hasn't been a new mother in Bellevue in the last twenty years who's given her baby the attention that this one's gotten."

"But my God," I yelled in exasperation. "What the hell are those two going to do to a little boy?"

"Frankly, I shudder to think," the social worker said. "But you might as well calm down. There's nothing you can do about it. You just can't set right all the wrongs in this world, so why don't you just relax, and act like a doctor instead of a social worker."

The next morning, as I stood by and advanced my day of total baldness, Charlene and Paula took their baby home. Since then, I've often wondered what became of him. Probably in a few years I'll be watching him play tackle for the Los Angeles Rams.

Now that homosexuality has gone public, the peculiar medical problems attending the condition are also better known, and so homosexuals probably receive better care than they did fifteen years ago. But I'll bet that plenty of them still get their treatment at The Vue. Depending upon the eyes of the beholder, gay may be beautiful, but it still has a way to go before it can claim to be a truly accepted way of life.

6

Marriages Are Made in Heaven

One of the most intriguing things about working at Bellevue was the manner in which we were repeatedly shown how stupid we were. Although most of us had left medical school with a good grounding in treating various diseases and with a fine appreciation for the scientific method, very few of us knew how to listen intelligently to what our patients were telling us. This knack eventually came with experience, but before we had learned our lesson, we often managed to make ourselves look very silly.

The problem of marital disputes was unconditionally guaranteed to provide an inexperienced physician every opportunity to make a fool of himself. Students and residents on obstetrics and gynecology were especially susceptible to this snare, since difficulties related to the reproductive system frequently led the complainant across a very tenuous line into a discussion of the problems of her married life.

For example, the ever-patient and long-suffering wife of the drunkard was a classic situation at The Vue. "What in the world am I going to do?" the patient would ask us, as the stereotyped tears began to form a puddle in her lap. "My husband goes to the bar every payday, and the money he doesn't spend on booze he gambles away. Then when I tell him they shut off the phone because we didn't have the money to pay the bill, he beats me up."

We thought the answer was obvious. "Admit your mistake," we advised. "Get a divorce from him. Start fresh. Profit from your mistake."

We really should have known better. For many years wiser heads than our own had been correctly diagnosing these interpersonal relationships. If any of us had bothered to read George Ade's

Fable of Flora and Adolph and a Home Gone Wrong, we'd have saved ourselves a good deal of trouble and embarrassment. The little story of Mr. and Mrs. Botts's day in divorce court would have taught us that marriages are indeed made in heaven, and that it is not for us to interfere.

But in our ignorance and innocence, we almost invariably rushed in foolishly, as a number of us did in the case of Adelina Hernandez. Adelina was a cute little nineteen-year-old with a thirty-five-year-old husband. At the time she and I became acquainted, she had just delivered her first baby and was ready to be checked over before being discharged. I examined her and found everything to be in working order, whereupon I gave her the usual going-home instructions. These included no intercourse for six weeks; at that one, she covered her mouth with her hand and giggled. Then the nurse began to tell her about feeding and bathing the baby, and I went on to check the next patient.

I didn't give Adelina another thought until she showed up late that same evening. The aide from the A.O. wheeled her in. Her face was swollen and suffused with tears, and she was pressing a bloody turkish towel against her nether regions. I asked her what had happened.

She managed to hold back the snuffling and sobbing long enough to choke out, "My husbin', he done it."

I put her up on the examining table and looked. Then I groaned. Her repaired episiotomy—my beautiful work of art— was gaping wide open, with threads of catgut suture hanging out here and there. Deep in the base of the crater, a large vein oozed lazily but steadily.

"Your . . . husband?" I asked. "But why?"

"I dunno," she wailed. "He jes' say he's my husbin' and he ain't gonna wait no six weeks."

I called Vince Ciccone, the senior resident, and repeated the story to him. Vince came down to the floor, inspected the casualty, and began muttering quietly to himself. He sutured the bleeding vessel shut, and then sat for a moment, reevaluating the situation.

"It looks clean," he said. "Let's close it again." He put a new layer of gut stitches into the wound, after which he waved his index finger at Adelina.

"No more *contacto*," he growled. *"Comprende?"*

Adelina nodded her head.

Vince motioned me to leave the room with him. "I've seen this happen before," he said out of the corner of his mouth. "Usually the bleeding scares the shit out of the husband, and it's months before he'll go near her again."

"Good," I said, and we proceeded to forget about Adelina—at least until the following night, when she turned up at The Vue again in pretty much the same condition as the night before, except that she wasn't bleeding quite as heavily. This time, my senior resident on call was Bud Romansky. Bud came down to the floor, sewed up Adelina's bottom, and then proceeded to deliver a lecture to her, describing the horrors of infection in vivid detail. Adelina was shaking as she went out the door.

Nevertheless, she was back again the following evening. Tears, wailing, and ripped-out suture material were all carbon copies of the previous two nights. Wearily I stuffed a gauze pad into her traumatized perineum and called Vince Ciccone, who was back on service for the night.

When Vince stormed into the examining room, Adelina was sending heart-rending Ay's heavenward, and the nurse was clucking over her, saying words of comfort interspersed with curses directed against that sex maniac of a husband of hers. Vince unceremoniously ripped out the gauze I had put in to slow the bleeding and stared for a moment at the gaping crater. "Jee-sus Christ," he roared. "I'm gonna fix that son-of-a-bitch." He turned to the nurse. "Get me some number 0 wire sutures," he said.

Then Vince proceeded to sew together the deeper layers of the episiotomy with catgut, as usual, but when he came to repair the lining of the vaginal wall, he used the wire, cutting each stitch so as to leave a line of sharp little barbs running the length of the vagina. Then he stood up and sighed contentedly.

"Okay, Mama," he said to Adelina. "Now, you go on home. But you've got to come back to the Clinic in ten days for me to take out these stitches—you got that?"

Adelina, as usual, nodded.

The next night I got a phone call from the Admitting Office. Chuck Markowitz, the urology resident, wanted me to come down for a minute. "Thought you might like to see the fruits of your labor," he said.

When I walked into the room, Chuck greeted me with a grin. "You got him," he said. "I'll say one thing for you OB guys: you sure do know how to make the punishment fit the crime."

Chuck was working on a guy who was gritting his teeth just as hard as he could; periodically he would fling his head sharply from one side to the other. He was covered with sheets from his chest to his knees, with his penis protruding through a little hole cut at the proper level. At least I assumed it was his penis; it looked more like a skinny, raw meat loaf. Chuck was dabbing at it with antiseptic, applying minute dressings, and occasionally carefully placing an ultrafine suture through one of the deeper, bloodier gashes.

Pausing for a moment, Chuck looked back at me over his shoulder. "It's a miracle he missed cutting the urethra," he said. "Then we'd have had a repair job and a half on our hands before he'd ever pee again."

Just watching was making my groin twitch sympathetically. "Looks bad enough to me, urethra or not," I said.

"Oh, he'll feel this for a good long while," said Chuck. "Long enough, I'd say, for that episiotomy to heal up."

I walked the few steps to the head of the table. "What do you say, Mr. Hernandez?" I intoned righteously. "You think you can manage to leave Adelina alone now for a few days?"

Hernandez focused his bloodshot eyes on me. "Yeah, I guess so," he muttered.

That wasn't good enough for me. "What's the matter with you, anyway?" I said. "You ought to know you've got to stay away from your wife after she's had a baby."

"Aw, come on, Doc," he whined. "I'm not a bad guy; I knew that. But you know what that li'l bitch was doin' to me?" His eyes flashed with anger, and suddenly his voice lost its peevish quality, the tone becoming one of injured pride. "She went and put on her nightgown, one o' them things you can see through, and then she began makin' fun of me, telling me I couldn't have any for six whole weeks. Well, that was enough to give me a pretty good hard-on, but I still didn't do nothing; I didn't even touch her. So what'd she go an' do?"

I shook my head from side to side, although I had a pretty good idea of what she had gone and did. I was beginning to have a terrible feeling of remorse in the pit of my stomach.

"I'll tell yuh," said Mr. Hernandez. "She came over to me and started rubbing her tits against me, and then she jammed her cunt—excuse me, Doc, but that's what she did—into my knee. Then she started kissing me on the neck and all over the place— well, I'll tell you—"

I don't think I've ever seen another man so angry. For a moment I was afraid he was going to jump off the table.

"—God damn, she *is* my wife, and I wasn't gonna let her get away with shit like that. I figured, that's the way she wants it, that's okay with me. Y' understand what I mean, Doc?"

"Yeah," I said. "I understand."

Chuck had stopped working during the monologue, and now he was staring malevolently at me.

"You bastards!" he hissed.

I walked quietly out the door, and back up to the obstetrics floor.

Happily, I never saw either Hernandez again, but did I learn from my experience? Only a few months later one of our patients appeared for her weekly examination in the prenatal clinic, about two weeks before she was due to deliver. She looked as though she had been used for first base in the seventh game of the World Series. Her face was cut and bruised, one eye was tightly shut, and her body and extremities were a mass of black-and-blue blotches. I asked what had happened to her.

"Mah huzbin' done beat me up las' night," she drawled. Then she favored me with her shy ear-to-ear grin.

I had known this woman for several weeks, and I had long since concluded that she was the most blatantly stupid patient I had ever treated. She was seventeen, and had come to us courtesy of her twenty-four-year-old husband, a welfare recipient, who had impregnated her during one of his visits back to his little home town in southern Alabama. Then he had made an honest imbecile out of her. When I had first seen her in the Clinic, I had thought that she was beginning to retain too much fluid, so I told her to avoid salt. A week later, she was five pounds heavier, but she said she had indeed avoided salt. So I asked her what she had had for supper the previous evening.

"Hot doags," she answered with her oligophrenic smile. "An' peets-uh. Then ah hayd sum popcohn fo' dee-zuht."

I tried to explain that these foods were loaded with salt, but she objected: "Waal, ah dint *ayid* enny salt, jes' lahk y' said." So there.

At that point, I gave her a spelled-out, salt-free diet. When she returned the following week, I asked her whether she had stuck to the diet. She said she had. "Did you like it?" I asked. She said she had indeed.

Now I thought I had her. Any person who admits she likes a salt-free diet must be cheating; the food has all the taste appeal of well-soaked blotting paper. But then I looked at her chart and discovered she had lost eight pounds during the week. The girl was so stupid that she not only had stuck to a salt-free diet, but had actually liked it. I suppressed the urge to sprinkle salt on her head to see whether she would dissolve like a slug, and went on to the next patient.

Thus it went for several weeks until the current episode. I quickly made the decision that it would be best to keep her in protective custody in the hospital until she delivered, and I so advised her. She—what else?—smiled.

That girl was the sensation of the maternity ward. The nurses took one look at her and turned pale. They shrieked aloud about what kind of animal her husband must have been, and proceeded to shower her with attention and tenderness. Later that afternoon, the head nurse came up to me. "She's such a sweet little thing, she crooned. "I'd sure like to get my hands on that husband of hers." I, however, allowed that after having seen what he was capable of doing to his wife, did not share the nurse's desire to get my hands on him.

That night the husband came to visit. He was a six-foot greaser, dressed in a zoot suit. He cruised around the ward, jollying and pinching the nurses, and then made his way into the ward kitchen, opened the refrigerator, and helped himself to some of our food. Then, restored in body and soul, he came to the desk, where he proceeded to thank me profusely for caring so well for his wife. "Ah'd lahk t' give yew a cee-gar," he said with a smirk, "but ah cain't afford it on mah welfare check." I assured him I appreciated the sentiment. Besides, I didn't smoke cee-gars anyway.

As he left the ward, he gave his wife a tender pat on the butt, and told her to be sure and mind all that the doctors and nurses told her. She, of course, smiled at him and nodded yes.

It was during rounds the next morning that the revelation came to me. I was in the middle of checking my little friend's abdomen when a question suddenly popped into my head. I really don't know why. Looking up at the girl, I asked her why it was that her husband had decided to beat up on her.

She flashed me her biggest smile. "Oh, ah jes' got tard o' havin' him alla time drinking down at the bar with his friends," she said calmly. "So, ah went aftuh him wif the biggest carvin' knife we got."

The head nurse, who was standing behind me, turned chalky

and staggered out of the room. I eased myself into the nearest chair and began to laugh. The girl, delighted at having been able to bring a little cheer into our day, beamed at me and added, "Ah reely wuz gonna kill 'im, too."

That episode finally caused me to become considerably more wary of accepting one person's stories of his or her marital woes. From that time on, I never felt the same when a patient told me a tearful tale about how her husband was drinking away the family food money, or how he had brought her a gift of a case of clap. I'd simply suggest that she go and seek the advice of a professional marriage counselor; I even began to make referrals. For my own part, I figured she might just as well go home and count her blessings. Undoubtedly, her marriage was made in heaven.

7

Things Ain't Always What They Seem

One night during my third year of medical school, I was covering the general pediatrics ward, and my hands were full to overflowing. The last thing in the world I needed or wanted right then was a new admission. Every bed was occupied; we had just admitted a baby with a hideous case of the galloping green shits, and there was more than the usual workbookful of general scut to be taken care of. I simply didn't have any time to spend on a new patient.

My heavy workload had lowered my mood about as far down as it ever goes. Nor did it help matters that I detested pediatrics. I couldn't wait to finish serving my time so I could get off the service, never to return. It was bad enough to have to watch those kids dying of some of the most dreadful diseases one could imagine, but on top of that I managed to catch every non-lethal illness they had to communicate. Both my nose and my intestines ran constantly. Furthermore, drawing blood samples on them was the nearest thing to being put on the rack: if they didn't spit on me, they peed on me; and if they managed to remain continent, they bit me. Worse than the patients were their bitching and bitchy mothers. I'd have preferred to serve my pediatrics clerkship shoveling out latrines.

Thus, I considered throwing in the towel when I saw the messenger wheel in a little girl and leave her at the nurses' desk. She appeared to be about three years old, had long blonde hair and the pallor of chronic illness. She wore a listless, sad expression. Her mother and father stood behind the chair, she biting her lower lip, and he picking at his fingernails. The three of them were dressed in plain, shabby garments. The child had generous smears of dirt around her mouth, and the father looked as though he delivered coal for a living, which he may well have done. I watched as Joel Gaylord, the intern, walked over and introduced himself. He scanned the admission slip, and then said, "What's the trouble with Rosie tonight?"

The father looked at the mother. She shrugged, and then, realizing that the burden of communication had been placed upon her, mumbled, "She don't feel so good."

"Well, don't worry," said Joel, using his most professionally reassuring voice. "We'll see what's bothering her." He looked in my direction, raised his voice, and called out, "Dr. Karp. Would you come here a minute, please?"

"Yes, Dr. Gaylord," I growled through my clenched teeth as I walked up to the little group.

"Dr. Karp, this is Mr. and Mrs. Murchison and little Rosie," said Joel, dripping oil all over my shoes. "I'd like you to take a history and check her over. When you're done, give me a call up in my room."

I felt utterly exasperated. "Joel, for God's sake," I said. "I still haven't cultured up that baby with diarrhea, and I've got a mountain of scut. Can't you just work this one up yourself?"

"One thing at a time, Dr. Karp, and I'm sure you'll get it all done by morning," pontificated Joel. "Besides," he added out of the corner of his mouth, "just remember: it's all a learning experience." With that, he took off down the hall.

As I watched him go, I silently prayed that his mattress would be infested with armies of hungry crotch crickets. Then I sighed, turned back to the Murchisons, and asked them to come with me into the little waiting room off the corridor leading to the ward. There we sat down, and I proceeded to pull teeth.

Getting a history out of these people was a truly frustrating assignment. The father proved to be totally non-verbal: his communication was limited to gestures and grunts. Rosie sat in the wheelchair, stared blankly into space, and appeared to not even hear the questions I put to her. That left only the mother, a retiring little woman whose speech, like her dress, conveyed the extreme poverty of her lifelong environment. But at least she talked.

By keeping the questions brief and straightforward, I was able to learn that for the past few months Rosie had been behaving oddly. There had been stretches of time during which she had seemed perfectly all right, but at increasingly frequent intervals she had been acting irritable and drowsy. In addition, her appetite was failing. Four days previously, she had caught a severe cold that the mother claimed had been in circulation among all the neighborhood children. Then, for the past two days, she had been vomiting and complaining of headache.

"Has she had any fever?" I asked. Specters of meningitis danced in my mind.

"No, I've been taking her temperature all the time. She's been acting so funny," the mother said. "But even when she had the cold so bad last Monday, there wasn't no fever."

"What made you bring her in tonight?" I asked. "She's been sick, you say, for about three months. Did something special happen tonight?"

For the first time, the mother seemed animated. "Oh yes, Doctor. Tonight, I knew we had to bring her in. About two hours ago it was, she was standing right in front of me when she got this funny look on her face and her eyes rolled way up, and then she fell down on the floor and had a fit, you know, shaking her arms and legs back and forth."

"Did she bite her tongue?" I asked. "Or wet her pants?"

"Well, I did see a little blood coming out of her mouth afterwards," replied the mother. "And she went pottty, like you said, right on the rug."

About this time I began to feel very sad. The mother had given me a classic history for a brain tumor, and brain tumors in children are usually highly malignant and beyond surgical cure by the time they manifest themselves. My physical examination didn't make me feel any better. Rosie's pulse rate was very slow, and when I looked into her eyes with an ophthalmoscope, there was obvious swelling around the optic nerve, a sign of increased pressure within the brain. These, too, were findings suggestive of a brain tumor.

I called Joel, and he came down and checked my findings. He agreed with the grim diagnosis and prognosis. "But we ought to do a spinal tap," he said. "If there's increased protein or an elevated number of lymphocytes in the fluid, that would just about clinch it."

We did the tap. A short while later, the night emergency lab reported a protein content that was twice normal and ten times as many lymphocytes as there should have been. My depression reached an unprecedented low.

Rosie had been put into a bed with side rails, and I went back to the waiting room to talk to Mr. and Mrs. Murchison. Briefly, I outlined the findings. "It looks very much as though she's got something growing in her head," I said.

Mr. Murchison just continued to sit there, picking at his fingernails. Mrs. Murchison asked me whether that was bad.

"It's not good," I said.

"Can you get her better, Doctor?"

"I'm sorry," I said, "I really don't know for sure now. We're going to run some more tests in the next few days to see how big the growth is and where it's located. Then we'll be able to tell if we can get it out with an operation." I considered the fact that I had only five more weeks to spend on pediatrics; if I was lucky, Rosie would last beyond that time, and I wouldn't have to preside over her demise.

Mrs. Murchison wrung her hands. "I want to talk to you every day, Doctor," she said. "Are you here about five o'clock in the afternoon?"

I told her I would be available at that time. "But maybe you'd rather speak to Dr. Gaylord," I suggested. "He's actually in charge of my work."

The woman shook her head. "You're her doctor," she said, "so I want to talk to you." That was that. Lucky me.

The next morning, Joel and I made rounds with Charlie Evers, the resident. I presented Rosie's case to him. He nodded, checked out her physical findings, and said um-hum. "You're sure you're not overlooking anything," he added. "Could she have meningitis? Or encephalitis? Or even a brain abscess?"

"Not likely on the first two without fever and more signs of neurologic impairment," Joel said. "And it's a pretty chronic course for a brain abscess. But if she does have one, the tests we're ordering for brain tumor will show it up."

"How about a subdural hematoma?" asked Charlie. (That's a blood clot beneath the skull, on the surface of the brain.)

"I doubt that too," said Joel. "There's no history whatever of a head injury. And she's been sick pretty long for a subdural. Also, the routine skull films we got last night don't show anything suggestive."

"Okay," Charlie said. "What are you going to do next?"

"She's scheduled for an angiogram today," Joel replied. "We got her on as a special case."

Rosie went for her angiogram that afternoon. The radiologists injected a dye into the arteries leading to her brain, and then took X-rays. The blood vessels which nourish brain tumors show a characteristic arrangement. But Rosie's angiogram was entirely normal.

This did not completely rule out a brain tumor, however, and Joel and I scheduled Rosie for her next test, a pneumoencephalogram. This involves the injection of air into the central fluid-filled cavity of the brain. Then, more X-rays are taken to determine whether there is any displacement of the normal contours of the air space. This test is more difficult and more dangerous than an angiogram, and by the time the sweating neuroradiologists had completed their work, more than two hours had passed, and Rosie had another negative test to her credit.

Mrs. Murchison clasped her hands together as I told her the news. "Oh, I'm awful glad, Doctor," she said softly. "I don't want anything to be growing in Rosie's head. Do you think she'll be okay now?"

"I really don't know," I answered. "We still thinks she has a growth, but maybe it's located where the X-rays don't show it up." Translated, that meant right smack in the middle of her brain tissue, but I couldn't quite say that. "We'll go over her case again in the morning and see what else we might be able to do."

Meanwhile, Rosie's clinical course had been none too reassuring. She was becoming increasingly unresponsive and lethargic, and since she had been in the hospital, she had had two further convulsions. After the first one, we had started her on phenobarbital to try to forestall any further seizures, but obviously we had not had much success.

In the morning, as we reached Rosie's bed, Charlie reexamined the child and then thumbed slowly through the chart, pausing to study the laboratory results. "Are you absolutely sure she has a brain tumor?" he asked.

"There's nothing else she *could* have," Joel answered. I nodded my head in agreement.

Charlie um-hummed and turned back to Rosie. He opened her mouth and pulled her lower lip away from the gum. "What's this?" he asked sharply.

Joel and I peered into the crevasse. Running the length of the gum, right below the line of tooth insertions, was a black line. I had no idea what it was.

Joel whistled. "Jee-sus Christ!" he said. "Is that a lead line?"
"Looks like it to me," said Charlie. "Better get to work."

We got to work. Before the day was over, we had established that Rosie had elevated levels of lead in her blood and her urine, increased density at the ends of the bones of her legs, and peculiar blue dots in her red blood cells. Taken together, all these findings were diagnostic of chronic lead poisoning.

Lead poisoning, or plumbism, is a disease far more likely to be encountered at The Vue than at private institutions because of the way in which it's usually contracted. It is an environmental disease. Until recent years, most paints were compounded with a lead base so that when the paint began to peel off a wall and found its way into a small child's mouth the kid would slowly absorb the lead from its gut and suffer the disastrous consequences. Not only were the Bellevue pediatric clientele at greater risk because peeling walls in their tenement homes were less likely to be repaired, but in addition, some pediatricians have expressed the opinion that the poor diet to which the children were characteristically exposed made them more likely to want to eat the paint.

Rosie's course was typical of lead poisoning. Unfortunately, the disease tends to mimic other conditions which occur more frequently and which are, therefore, better known. As in Rosie's case, it can appear as an encephalitis with many of the signs of the various disorders we had in fact considered. Alternatively, the major symptom may be colic, in which case a number of abdominal diseases can be imitated. In either event, lead poisoning will be diagnosed only if the doctor keeps its possibility in mind.

If Joel and I hadn't been wearing blinders, we might have paused when we noticed how low Rosie's red blood cell count was. This too is typically found in plumbism. But we were convinced she had a brain tumor, so we simply ascribed the anemia to her poverty-level diet and to the lack of appetite characteristically seen in patients with brain tumors. Fortunately, Charlie Evers' mind remained open; he made the connection and looked for the black lead staining on the gums that I had simply chalked up to poor hygiene. Similarly, the basophilic stippling, or blue dots, on Rosie's smeared-out red blood cells hadn't impressed us. When you're absolutely certain the diagnosis is a brain tumor, it's easier to write off any discordant data than to try to interpret them.

Lead poisoning is a dangerous disease. One quarter to one half of the patients who appear with encephalitic symptoms die, and many of the survivors are mentally retarded, paralyzed, or suffer recurrent seizures. The effect of the lead on the nerve cells of the brain is devastating. All one can do is treat and hope for the best.

The therapy is directed toward two goals: preventing any further absorption of lead into the body and accelerating excretion of the lead that has already been taken up.

Absorption is prevented by removing all sources of ingestible lead from the environment and by feeding large quantities of milk, which converts the lead into a non-absorbable form. Excretion is accomplished by giving the patient ethylenediamine tetra-acetic acid (EDTA), a chemical which binds lead to itself and then carries it out in the urine. Toxic levels of lead in tissues and blood are further reduced by the administration of large quantities of calcium, phosphorus, and Vitamin D. These agents lower the solubility of lead in the bloodstream and augment its rate of deposition in bone, where it causes no harm.

All three of us on the ward house staff were considerably distressed over the missed diagnosis because in the two-day interval Rosie's condition had worsened. She now lay quietly in her bed, unaware and unresponsive. This suggested that there was considerable swelling of the brain tissues, and that if she were to be saved, absolutely no further time could be lost. We decided to pass a tube into her stomach, pour milk through it, and at the same time, give her injections of calcium, phosphorus, and Vitamin D. Joel said he'd get right over and set up an intravenous infusion of EDTA.

"Isn't there something you want to do first?" asked Charlie.

Joel looked puzzled. I was puzzled.

"If she does have any lead left in her intestines, the EDTA'll make it more absorbable, and that would worsen her symptoms." Charlie pounded his fist into his hand. "We've got to get a film of the abdomen and see whether there's still any lead in her gut."

"I know we're giving her the milk, just to be on the safe side," said Joel. "But she's been out of her house for two days already. Do you really think she's got any lead left inside? It seems like a wasted X-ray."

"You were sure she had a brain tumor, too," said Charlie dryly.

Joel wrote out the requisition for the X-ray. It turned out that it *was* negative for lead in the gut, but he didn't complain.

For each of the next five days, either Joel or I gave Rosie an intravenous infusion of EDTA, and at least twice a day we reviewed her neurological status. By the fourth day, when I pinched the little girl, she made an effort to move away and let out a high-pitched groaning noise. On the day after that her eyes periodically flickered open.

It's safe to give EDTA for only five days at a stretch, so during the next two days, Rosie received no chemical therapy. We all held our breath and watched her. Fortunately, she continued to improve. Our treatment must have mobilized a large quantity of lead from her blood and her tissues. On the seventh day, she shakily tried to sit up in bed. But in the same day, the lead concentration in her blood, which had been falling, showed a slight increase. This indicated that the metal remaining in her body was not being excreted fast enough, and so, beginning the next morning, we initiated a second course of EDTA therapy. The blood lead level fell immediately, and after the drug was again discontinued did not rise.

After Rosie had spent four weeks in The Vue, she was ready to go home. She had recovered neurologically, except for a slight residual weakness of her left arm. Her parents, who came each day to visit her, were sufficiently impressed to declare that Charlie, Joel, and I were, without question, genuine incarnations of Our Savior. At least, so the mother declared, and the father nodded in vigorous agreement.

Before we discharged Rosie, we took care to tell her parents that it was very important for us to see her regularly in the clinic so that we might monitor her continued progress. In addition, as tactfully as he could, Charlie warned Mr. and Mrs. Murchison that there are often long-term sequelae of lead encephalitis, including mental retardation due to damage to the brain cells. It was like talking to the wall. Mrs. Murchison replied that she "just knew" there wouldn't be anything wrong. Mr. Murchison hugged his daughter and murmured over and over, "My little Rosie." I realized that those were the first words I had ever heard him speak.

We sent out one of the social workers to make certain Rosie would get her necessary follow-up, and also to check the home situation. She returned in a grand snit.

"You just can't imagine that place," she said. "Two rooms, three kids, all kinds of crap all over the place, and strips of paint six inches long peeling off the wall. I showed the paint to the Murchisons and told them that was how Rosie got sick, and that she'd get sick again if they didn't fix the place up."

"So what'd they say?" I asked.

"Mrs. Murchison said they knew all that, because you guys had told them the same thing while Rosie was in the hospital," said the social worker. "She said they'd been working on the landlord to scrape and paint, but he told them he wasn't about to do that for the amount of rent they paid. He also said that he thought what they had was good enough for slobs like them. So Mr. Murchison led me over to one of the closets, opened it up, and showed me a couple of cans of paint, a brush, and a scraper. His wife said he was going to do the job this weekend.

Mr. Murchison did the job, the family received some dietary counseling, and that was the end of the lead poisoning in that household. Unfortunately, however, there were thousands of other people in New York living under similar conditions, so plumbism remained a recurring problem among the Bellevue pediatric population. Its importance has not declined with time, despite the fact that increasing numbers of tenements have been repainted with the newer leadless paints, in compliance with the 1959 New York City law. There has been no significant improvement because the original layers of paint remain under the new ones, as toxic as ever. Thus, even today, most of the poorly fed toddlers in the Bellevue catchment area still can't gnaw the peelings off their walls without running the risk of developing lead poisoning.

8

The Healing of John the Baptist

Throughout its history, Bellevue Hospital has numbered very few famous persons among its patients. The fact of the matter is that a huge municipal hospital catering to the Lower East Side of New York, with its open wards, its peeling plaster, and its rats and roaches offers very little to attract the ailing celebrity crowd. However, fame and insolvency are not mutually exclusive traits, and so there have been occasional exceptions to the rule.

For example, in the winter of 1864 a thirty-eight-year-old alcoholic was brought to The Vue from his flophouse, where he had passed out. He was suffering from pneumonia, a lethal disease in those pre-penicillin days, especially when it attacked a malnourished derelict such as this one. The man lived for only three days. In his pocket, the attendants found thirty-eight cents and a scrap of paper on which were written the words, "Dear friends and gentle hearts." Music students later concluded that this was to have been the first line of a song that the man had intended to write. He was composer Stephen Foster.

Exactly one hundred years later, as a Bellevue intern, I took care of a luminary of even greater renown. Let the former interns at Los Angeles' Cedars-Sinai brag about the actresses for whom they were called to prescribe sleeping pills late at night when no one would dare to rouse a private physician. Let the erstwhile house officers at Columbia University's Harkness Pavilion boast of the political dignitaries who once upon a time deigned to permit them to draw samples of blood. None of these doctors has anything on me.

Not one of them can make the claim I can: for ten days I served as personal physician to John the Baptist.

John came under my care on a bitterly cold January night. The radiators were hissing and were giving off little jets of steam. I was at the desk, near the front of the ward, reviewing the day's lab slips while my wife transcribed them into the charts. Nearby, the ward clerk and the messenger were playing gin. I heard the elevator door clang down the long stone hallway. A minute later I looked up to see the Admitting Office messenger wheel in an old man in a wheelchair.

The new patient was about six feet tall, but he couldn't have weighed more than a hundred and twenty pounds. He had long, gray hair and a beard, and both looked as though they hadn't been combed in more than a year. His eyes were little and abnormally bright, and the way they were darting all around the room put me in mind of a sparrow on a telephone wire. He didn't smell like a sparrow, though: his odor would have shamed a full-grown billy goat. In one hand he clutched a worn, dirty Bible, and in the other he held a straight, three-foot-long stick. All in all, he looked like a sick and dissipated John Brown.

I got up and walked over to the man. "How do you do, sir," I said. "I'm Dr. Karp. What's your name?"

"John the Baptist," said my new patient weakly. Before I could react he lifted his stick and began to wave it in my direction. "Do you believe in the Lord Jesus Christ?" he demanded to know.

I cogitated for a very brief moment, and then answered, "Yes sir, I certainly do."

The old man dropped his stick back into his lap and rumbled, "Very well, then, I will not fear."

"Good," I said. "Now, tell me: is John the Baptist your real name, or is that just what you call yourself?"

"Why, my real name, of course."

At that point I took the admission slip from the messenger, who headed off at top speed down the hallway, dramatically holding his nose and pretending that he was about to become violently sick to his stomach. According to the official hospital document, the patient's name was Baptist, John; he had no known address; and his admitting diagnosis was "RLL pneum." This was an abbreviation for pneumonia of the lower lobe of the right lung, a very common cause for admission of these elderly, emaciated, often alcoholic gentlemen during the New York winter season.

"Let's try once more," I said, and looked into John's eyes. "Are you the original John the Baptist, or a reincarnation? Or are you a guy whose name happens to be John Baptist?"

The old fellow looked annoyed. He glared up at me and said, very slowly, as though he were addressing a child, "My . . . name . . . is . . . John . . . the . . . Baptist."

That settled that. At least I knew he had a middle name.

"How did you get here?" I asked.

"I don't know."

The admitting paper said he had been found by a policeman, helpless on the sidewalk. Again, the usual Bellevue winter's tale.

"What's bothering you, John?" I said.

"I have a great pain here." He pointed to his right lower rib cage. "My very breath itself causes pain."

I assured him we'd take care of his problem very shortly, and then set about working him up. The physical examination, the blood count, the appearance of his sputum, all were characteristic of bacterial pneumonia. To be certain of the extent of the disease, and to be sure there was no tuberculosis underlying the pneumonic infection, I sent him down for X-rays. My wife wheeled him away and I wrote up his chart and his orders.

Forty-five minutes later she wheeled him back, carrying a huge sheaf of X-rays under her arm.

"My God, what took you so long?" I asked.

Myra pushed the wheelchair a little distance away and then came over to whisper to me. "They had to take three shots for every one you ordered. Whenever they told him to stop breathing and move, he'd start waving that stick and call the wrath of God down on the heads of all disbelievers."

"Oh."

"Then, finally, the X-ray tech just lost all her patience with his moving around. She shoved him against the machine and hollered at him, 'God damn it, now, hold still, you stupid old bastard.' That didn't set too well with your friend."

I closed my eyes and ground my teeth. "No, I guess he wouldn't have taken too kindly to that," I said.

"That's putting it mildly," replied my wife. "He went after her with the stick, yelling something or other about smiting the sinners as did Isaiah in the days of yore. I finally managed to get him calmed down and made him stand still long enough to take the pictures."

I looked at John. He was slumped in his wheelchair, his head lolling above the right armrest. I went over and checked him. Sure enough, his temperature had gone up from 101° to almost 104°, and his pulse was disturbingly fast and weak. So I put him to bed, gave him aspirin to lower the fever, and started an intravenous infusion of penicillin solution. After this, I checked the X-rays: they revealed the presence of a severe pneumonia, but there was no evidence of tuberculosis. Then I returned to John's bedside for a moment. He was lying unconscious, breathing in and out thirty times a minute (approximately twice the normal rate), the whiskers near his mouth moving back and forth with the breeze.

"Is he going to make it?" Myra whispered from behind me.

I shook my head. "Can't really tell for twenty-four hours or so. All we can do is hook him up to the antibiotics and hope." I checked my watch; it was eleven o'clock. I decided it was time to get some sleep.

When my phone rang, my watch read a quarter to five. I snapped the receiver off the hook and growled a hello.

"Dr. Karp?" It was the night nurse on the ward.

"Yeah," I growled. Interns always hope that night calls will turn out to be wrong numbers.

"Listen, Dr. Karp. You'd better come on down to the ward. Mr. John the Baptist pulled out his intravenous needle, and he's causing a terrible ruckus here."

"Oh, God. I'll be right over."

The entrance to the long, rectangular Bellevue wards was occupied by a nurses' desk, and on one side were medication cabinets, with examination rooms on the other. The rest of the ward space was taken up by three rows of about fifteen beds each, two rows down each wall and one down the middle. According to the custom, as the newest, sickest admission, John the Baptist was occupying the bed nearest the nursing station. He was sitting up, his beard and his hair flying in all directions, and he was waving his stick. The smashed penicillin bottle lay at the foot of the bed, and blood dripped from his arm where the needle had been. His shrill voice pierced the semidarkness. "Beware, ye sinners, for the end of the world is near at hand. Thus saith the Lord."

The night nurse trotted over to me. "His temperature broke about an hour ago, Dr. Karp," she said. "Since then, he's been raising hell. He's got the whole place awake."

"Oh, Christ!"

"What are you going to do?"

"I don't know." I really didn't, either.

"We could bug him over to psych."

"No, we don't want to do that."

"Why not?"

"Because the intern on that ward weighs thirty pounds more than I do, and he'd kill us both if we dumped this mess on him at five o'clock in the morning."

Meanwhile, the sermon went on. "The meek shall inherit the earth," hollered John. "An eternity in the most fiery of hells awaiteth the sinner. Thus spake the Lord of Hosts."

"Shut up, you goddamnsonofabitch!" The command came straight from the heart of the Bowery denizen across the way, and it was punctuated by a flying metal urinal that bounced off the wall behind John, showered plaster all over him, and then fell to the tile floor with an ear-splitting clatter.

John looked up at the ceiling. "Oh Lord, Lord, deliver me from the hands of mine enemies," he implored. "Visit the wrath of Sodom and Gomorrah on the sinners."

Suddenly I had a magnificent idea. "That's it," I whispered. "That's the ticket." I pounded the poor night nurse on the back so hard that she stumbled forward, almost falling on her face.

"That's what?" she asked as she straightened up. But I didn't answer her; I was on my way over to John's bedside. As I drew near, John saw me coming and he lifted up his stick as if in preparation to part my hair. I was scared silly, but I tried not to show it.

"John!" I said.

He stopped in mid-swing, the stick poised over his head.

"Put down that stick, John," I commanded. "You dare not strike an angel of the Lord."

He looked at me as though I were some special sort of nut. "*What* say you?" he asked.

"The Lord is pleased with your work, John," I rapidly continued. "But the sinners do not heed your warnings."

"They will pay for their sins in the fiery furnaces of Shadrach, Meshach, and Abednego."

"But, John, the Lord desireth not the death of the sinner, but that he return to the way of righteousness and live. Thus, it is the will of the Lord that you visit purgatory, the better that you may tell the sinners the error of their ways."

John actually dropped his stick. "You mean . . . this is—"

"Yes, John. You must spend ten days and nights here. I have been commanded to guide you through. Then, when you are finished, you will go again among the sinners and make them see the true light."

John shot a glance at the guy who had thrown the urinal at him. "But that blasphemer over there—"

"John," I hissed. "That's an evil spirit. He's a demon, sent by Satan himself to make certain that you will fail, so that all the souls will come to him. But he cannot succeed. The Lord will make you stronger than your enemy."

John sat there, staring silently at me.

"John, you must not hesitate," I said. "Think of all the souls that will be lost if you defy the word of the Lord."

John the Baptist turned his fanatical gaze on me, and I tried hard to mirror it back. I must have proved I was as buggy as he, because he grasped my arm, closed his eyes, looked skyward, and called out, "O Master! As you suffered the pain of the cross for our sins, so will I suffer the tortures-of purgatory for the souls of my fellow men. I shall heed the call of my Lord."

I let out a deep breath, and told John that his faith would certainly please the Lord. Then I put the needle back into his arm, the nurse hung up a new bottle of penicillin, and we all went back to sleep.

For the next couple of days John the Baptist behaved himself and appeared to be convalescing smoothly. On the morning of the third day, though, we had a bit of tension when John waved his stick at one of the attending physicians who wanted to examine him while he was reading the Bible. We told the doctor that he'd have no trouble if he would only preface his examination with, "The Lord is my Strength and my Redeemer," one of John's favorite lines. The attending said he'd be damned first, and asked why didn't we just take the stick away. I explained we couldn't possibly do that; that it would convince John that the forces of evil had triumphed over him.

"Besides," said one of the residents with a smirk, "it was a personal gift to him from Jesus."

At that point, the attending stormed off the ward muttering that he'd seen nutty things at Bellevue, but when the doctors acted nuttier than the patients, it was time for him to leave. Such is the case with nonbelievers.

On the fourth day, the nurse called me because John, having improved to the point where we could discontinue the intravenous penicillin, was refusing his twice-daily intramuscular injection of the antibiotic I hustled over to the ward.

Using his always-ready stick for emphasis, John informed me that in no way was he going to accept this latest visitation from hell. I directed his attention to the sadistically grinning bum next to him. "John," I said, "the forces of hell must not triumph. Think of the consequences if you ignore the Lord's command to you."

The fire came into John's eyes, and he fixed his stare on his neighbor. "You shall *not* defeat me," he bellowed. "You shall return in failure to your evil master, and submit to his fearful punishment."

The guy in the next bed turned pale and lit out for the men's room. John took his shot, and that was that.

As promised, by the tenth day, John was ready for discharge. He was all set to stride forth, but had to be convinced that the wheelchair was necessary so no lurking devils could trip him and break his leg. As he rode off, I asked him where I might hear him preaching the Gospel.

"At Forty-fifth and Broadway," he said. "That's where there are more sinners than any other place on Earth."

I wasn't inclined to argue.

A couple of weeks later, I actually did go to hear him. My wife told me maybe I shouldn't. "What'll you do," she asked, "if he sees you there and starts yelling that you're the Angel of Mercy himself? You'll both end up in the hatch together."

"We'll stay in the back," I said. "He won't even see us."

We did and he didn't. The wind was howling around the corners of the buildings, and the temperature was in the mid-twenties. Wrapped in a gray, herringbone coat which was two sizes too large, and was closed with only one button, John the Baptist addressed himself to a rapidly changing crowd of about twenty-five. He drew attention to the Bible in his left hand, threatened with the stick in his right, and all the while promised his listeners an eternity in a fiery hell.

"Sounds good t' me awn a night like this," chuckled the man standing next to me, as he stuffed his red cheeks full of hot dog. "What the hell makes these nuts go on, huh, buddy? Oughter put 'im away where he can't hurt no one." Then, the guy waddled down the street toward the Promised Land of Forty-second Street.

We stayed a bit longer, until the combination of cold winds, jeers from the crowd, and the faint aroma of sulfur combined to drive us off. As we left, we passed to his right. He aimed the stick at me, and my heart began to pound. Here it comes, I thought.

"Young man, you won't be able to walk away like this on Judgment Day." His eyes burned into mine, and I looked away.

"He doesn't even remember you," whispered my wife.

"Thank God," I whispered back.

From time to time, I would see John the Baptist on his corner, but he never did give any indication that he remembered me. But that's all right; celebrities are that way. I'll bet the actresses and the politicians never gave a second thought to the interns at Cedars and Harkness, either.

9

I'd Rather Be Lucky Than Good

Some people are born losers. Through hard work and long effort, others manage to achieve the status of losers. Still others have losing thrust upon them. Many Bellevue patients fit into all three categories.

Probably, the Bellevue losers had their functional origin in the Five-P Syndrome. The five P's stood for Piss-Poor Protoplasm, Poorly Put Together. Basically, this elegant terminology described the situation of a person who had had lifelong suboptimal nutrition on which was superimposed the sort of neglect and self-abuse which often accompanies an impecunious existence. Then, when the insults of advancing age were added, it took only a relatively minor illness to drop the final straw. At that point, all the efforts of the Bellevue personnel would be in vain, as things would go from bad to worse to worst. The downward spiral would be irreversible, complications would accumulate in a geometric fashion, and the patient would breathe his last with tubes in every orifice and machines of every description humming and clattering frantically. Although the doctors never failed to gloomily take stock and wonder where they might have gone wrong in their care, the whole process was really nobody's fault. It was not only a medical, but also a serious sociological problem.

No patient's story could possibly illustrate this situation as well as Sarah Rosenbaum's. Hers is the saddest tale of bad luck I have ever encountered or, for that matter could imagine. She might have been invented on a rainy Sunday afternoon by Theodore Dreiser. Perhaps she was Al Capp's model for Joe Bftxplk. If she had been a sports star, she wouldn't have lacked for nicknames. Rotten-luck Rosenbaum. Out-of-the-frying-pan-and-into-the-fire

Rosenbaum. For-the-want-of-a-nail-the-kingdom-was-lost Rosenbaum. Very definitely, somebody up there did not appear to like Mrs. Rosenbaum

The saga began one wet morning when Mrs. Rosenbaum, a plump sixty-eight-year-old widow, left her Lower East Side apartment to do a little food shopping. She wheeled her metal shopping cart in front of her and moved slowly. Between her stiff hips and her varicose veins, she was just a bit unsteady on her feet. She was being so careful to look ahead of her that she never did notice the paper bag directly under her feet. Her right foot came down on the bag, slid forward, and *wham*—Mrs. Rosenbaum was flat on her back.

When she woke up, she found herself being lifted into a meat wagon, one of the rectangular Bellevue ambulances that bore an unpleasant similarity in appearance to a butcher's truck. She never did find out who had called the thing. Maybe it had been the keeper of the shop in front of which she had fallen. These bloody bodies on the sidewalk really do kill business.

Mrs. Rosenbaum had suffered a badly cut scalp, and the ambulance attendants applied pressure to the bleeding wound. The meat wagon sped directly to the Bellevue Admitting Office.

Here, the surgical intern and resident attended to the new patient. Scalp wounds are funny things. There's very little tissue between skin and bone, so that when the scalp is torn away the underlying blood vessels over the skull are easily ripped, and bleed freely. Since they lie directly on the surface of the skull bones, they can't be clamped, so the only thing to do is to quickly suture the tear and then apply heavy pressure to it. But in the meanwhile, a lot of blood can be lost.

Mrs. Rosenbaum had already bled heavily before she reached the hospital. As the surgeons washed and sutured, they noticed with some dismay that the heavy bleeding was continuing. Their dismay increased as they considered her age and high blood pressure. If she were to lose too much blood too fast, she'd have been a very good candidate for a heart attack. So they called for a pint of blood, and began a transfusion as they continued their suturing. By the time the pint of blood had run in, they were finished. Then they spent the next few hours making certain that the patient's heart action and blood pressure remained normal. This done, they put Mrs. Rosenbaum to bed till the next day. In the morning they rechecked her neurological status and her skull X-rays. Everything was normal, so they congratulated Mrs. Rosenbaum on her good luck, and sent her home.

With good luck like that . . .

For a while Mrs. R. felt pretty well, perhaps just a little dizzy now and then. Her stitches came out with no trouble. But a month or so later she began to feel a little sick to her stomach, and before long, she began to vomit. Some days she had diarrhea as well. This distressing state persisted for a few weeks, and then one morning Mrs. Rosenbaum looked into her mirror and noticed that she was a bright shade of yellow. "Mein Gott, I look like a Chinaman," she muttered, and ran out to catch the First Avenue bus up to Bellevue.

Her diagnosis was not much of a problem for the internal medicine intern. "It's serum hepatitis," he told her. "Jaundice. An infection in your liver."

"Gewalt! From vhere do I get dis infeckshun?"

"Probably from the blood transfusion you had," answered the intern. "These germs live in some people's blood."

"So vhy'd d'nudnicks giff me blood mit joims?" wailed Mrs. Rosenbaum.

The intern gently explained that there were no tests that would have permitted identification of a contaminated sample of blood. He also briefly pondered the fact that it was not strange that the blood was infected, since at that time the city's blood banks accepted as donors any drug addict or bum who came in eager to trade his reasonable blood count for the price of a fix or a few bottles of cheap wine. What the hell. Business was business.

"So now vot den?" asked Mrs. Rosenbaum.

The intern explained that a few weeks' rest in the hospital and a good diet should fix her up as good as new. Mrs. Rosenbaum shook her head sadly and lowered herself into the wheelchair to ride up to her ward.

After a few weeks had passed, the house staff on Mrs. Rosenbaum's ward began to get concerned. The blood tests were showing no resolution of the hepatitis. Furthermore, Mrs. R. was, if anything, more yellow than ever. So the gastroenterologist was called, a needle was passed into Mrs. Rosenbaum's liver to take a biopsy, and the verdict of the Great Omniscient Pathologist was awaited.

It came the next day: subacute hepatitis. Actually, the intern had not lied to Mrs. Rosenbaum. Hepatitis usually does last only a few weeks, but occasionally, for reasons entirely unknown, the infection fails to resolve, and persists in an active state. As in Mrs. R.'s case, when the disease doesn't clear up within a few weeks, we call it subacute hepatitis. Then, if it lasts even longer, we change its name to chronic hepatitis. If we can't treat it, maybe we can confuse it. In any event, subacute and chronic hepatitis are very serious conditions.

The ward house staff met in consultation with the gastroenterologist, and further plans were formulated. It was decided to give Mrs. Rosenbaum steroids: these are drugs related to cortisone which have salutary effects on long-standing inflammatory diseases, such as rheumatoid arthritis. Hepatitis being an inflammatory disease, some attempts have been made to treat it with steroids. The results have been equivocal, but this was perceived as better than the unequivocally dead patients who had received no definitive therapy.

So Mrs. Rosenbaum began to take her steroids and, lo and behold, her yellow color began to fade and her blood tests improved. She was really getting better. The staff congratulated her on her good fortune. Mrs. Rosenbaum, however, regarded them with a somewhat jaundiced eye.

After about a month on steroids, one of the interns suddenly recalled that these drugs sometimes cause bleeding from the stomach. So he got Mrs. Rosenbaum to save a stool sample to test for blood. It was positive. So was the next sample. So was the one after that.

This caused no little consternation among the doctors. The miracle drug that was apparently bringing the (by now) chronic hepatitis under control was at the same time apparently producing bleeding from the stomach. This could be dangerous. But so could the hepatitis if it were once again allowed free rein. As the group contemplated the possibilities, one bright fellow had a great idea: maybe the bleeding was not being caused by the steroid drug. Maybe Mrs. Rosenbaum had another cause for her internal hemorrhaging. So they drew straws and the loser went off to tell Mrs. Rosenbaum what lay in store for her now. A sigmoidoscopy and then a barium enema X-ray. Should these prove negative, then an upper G.I. X-ray series.

For a sigmoidoscopy, a patient gets on a table and points her rear end at the ionosphere. A man stands behind her with a ten-inch-long metal tube, which he gradually inserts into her rectum. Then he and his associates look up into the tube. Generally this is called a pornographic, multiple X-rated movie, but when it is performed in a hospital by physicians, it is then considered socially acceptable behavior. Acceptable, that is, except to him or her who is being scoped. For the uninitiated, let me say that it feels as though a freeway were being constructed between the rectum and the belly button. In any event, Mrs. Rosenbaum's sigmoidoscopy failed to show a cause for her bleeding.

So on to the barium enema, a procedure which involves filling the rectum full of dye and then taking X-rays to look for any irregularity within. This was more revealing. The cause of the bleeding was apparent. Mrs. Rosenbaum didn't have to stop her steroids. She had cancer of the rectum.

Now came an even more spirited discussion among the members of the house staff. Between her hepatitis and her high blood pressure, Mrs. Rosenbaum was a poor surgical risk. However, not to operate was to abandon her fate to the whims of her cancer.

Once again the straws were passed around, and the holder of the short one trudged out to discuss the problem with Mrs. Rosenbaum. As tactfully as he could, he told her that she had a cancer in her rectum, but it did not appear to have spread, and seemed curable by appropriate surgery.

Mrs. R. seemed to accept the news philosophically. I suspect that by this time she had seen the handwriting. She sighed and shrugged, and then asked, "This soij'ry, it's gonna be a beg on mein stomach?" The intern figured out that she meant a colostomy, squirmed a little, and nodded. Mrs. Rosenbaum nodded back. That afternoon, she was transferred to the surgery ward.

She remained there for a week, while surgeons and anesthesiologists planned and plotted the procedures which would offer the patient the best possible chance of leaving the operating room alive. Then, after seventy-two hours of enemas and purgatives to empty the bowel, she was pronounced ready for surgery the next morning.

About five hours before the proposed operation, the intern was called to the ward. Mrs. R. was complaining of severe pain in her chest, was pale and clammy, and was gasping for breath. The cardiogram was a formality. She had suffered a severe heart attack. Without ado, she was returned to the medicine ward from whence she had come.

This was the point at which I personally entered Mrs.

Rosenbaum's life for the first time, although she had long since become a hospital legend in her own time. During the week she had spent on the surgery ward, I had become the intern on her medicine ward.

So now, as though chronic hepatitis, rectal cancer, and a heart attack were not enough, Mrs. Rosenbaum's misery was compounded by having a whole new crop of doctors to take care of her. She responded by becoming deeply depressed and totally negative.

She needed more than just medical treatment. I tried to tell her that in six weeks she'd go back for her operation and that this was only a temporary setback. "Hoo hah," said Mrs. Rosenbaum, stretching her arms forth so that the entire ward should hear her. "Me he tells about temp'rerry setbecks." Then she turned to face the wall.

I tried to cheer her up by bringing one of her former interns to see her. Mrs. Rosenbaum looked daggers at him, said, "Foist he desoits me, den he comes 'n' giffs me leckchizz." Once again, she turned to face the wall.

One of the gastroenterologists thought that a psychiatry consultation might be of help. The Shrink talked to Mrs. Rosenbaum for a while, and then wrote a nice note on the chart to the effect that Mrs. Rosenbaum had a "reactive depression," that anyone who had her problems was perfectly entitled to be depressed, and that maybe the gastroenterologist needed a psychiatry consultant.

As the days passed, Mrs. Rosenbaum became more and more withdrawn. Finally, she stopped eating. So I went to talk to her. "Mrs. Rosenbaum," I said. "You've got to eat. Your heart isn't going to get better if you don't eat."

I was ready for an argument or a so-what statement, but what came back was, "De food ain't kosheh."

"But Mrs. Rosenbaum, you've eaten the food all along. Why all of a sudden do you decide it's not kosher?"

"I never t'ought about it before."

I decided to play the game, so I called the rabbi. He came right up to talk to Mrs. Rosenbaum, and assured her that not only was she permitted to eat non-kosher food when she was sick, but that he would arrange for her to receive kosher food from the hospital kitchen.

"Dot's no good," she said. "De pots 'n' pens here ain't kosheh." That was that. She turned to the wall.

That evening my wife and I sat in the examining room, and I told her about Mrs. Rosenbaum, who by this time had not eaten a thing in the previous forty-eight hours. My wife asked why I didn't pass a stomach tube and force-feed her. I explained that the battle it would cause might well produce another heart attack. My wife thought for a moment, and then said, "I think I can get her to eat."

"Be my guest, I said.

My wife got up and walked over to Mrs. Rosenbaum. "Hello, Mrs. Rosenbaum," she said. "I'm Myra Karp."

Mrs. R. turned and looked my wife up and down. "You Dokteh Kahp's wife?"

Myra admitted to the fact.

Mrs. Rosenbaum focused on the white coat. "I seen you here before, but I didn't know you was Dokteh Kahp's wife. You a dokteh too?"

Myra explained that she was not a dokteh, but that she came to the hospital at night to keep me company and to help me out by doing laboratory work and filling out charts.

Mrs. Rosenbaum smiled. "Now dot's nize," she said. "Dot's rilly, rilly nize. At night you come to dis place, to be mit your husbin. Vot you do all day?"

"I'm a schoolteacher," said Myra.

"A scullteechuh! Vot grade you teach?"

Myra explained that she taught home economics—sewing and cooking. This led up to the direct attack. "Since my husband says you won't eat the food here," she said, "tomorrow night, I'm going to bring you a chicken. And it will not only be kosher, it will be *good.*"

Mrs. Rosenbaum's eyes lit up. I was astonished. First, I had seen her smile, and now I had seen her show some interest in something—even if it was only a boiled chicken. The old lady grabbed Myra by the arm, and cried, "You mean dot? You are rilly gonna bring me a suppeh tomorrow?"

"Yes, I mean it," said Myra. "But I want you to be here to eat it. My husband and the other doctors are worried about you, you don't eat anything. I can't bring you three meals a day, so you've got to do something."

"Ah, no problem," smiled Mrs. Rosenbaum. "De rebbe sez I kin eat food dot ain't kosheh if I'm sick. So, I eat a little—just enuf to keep alife, till you bring d' chicken." Then she turned toward me and hollered across the room, "You got such a wife, Dokteh Kahp, I hope you're grateful for it." She patted Myra on the head.

At that point I walked down to the staff dining room and brought up a plate of bread and butter and a glass of milk. Mrs. Rosenbaum devoured the whole thing while she had an animated conversation with my wife for the next hour. I filled in the charts.

Over the next five weeks Mrs. Rosenbaum remained cheerful and well-fed. She exclaimed loudly over the meals my wife brought her, and repeatedly remarked how nize it vus dot a wife should come be mit her husbin. Then, when my wife would tell her how much better she looked, she'd smile and really act as though she believed it. Actually, she looked lousy: yellow, pale, wasted, and old. But cheerful.

Finally it was time for the surgeons to try again. We arranged to keep Mrs. R. on our ward right up until the operation, so she wouldn't have to go for a veek mit strenjihs. The night before the procedure, she wasn't allowed to eat solid food, so my wife brought her some chicken soup. As she gratefully acknowledged receipt of her supper, she reached under the bed and, with a flourish presented my wife with a big ribboned box. Myra opened it. Inside were several aprons. My wife was speechless.

"Mrs. Rosenbaum," I said. "Where did you get the aprons?"

"Mein sohn," she answered proudly. "He voiks in a apron fect'ry. So I told him to get them for me to giff your wife, she should heff sump'n nize to use t' teach d' kids in."

"I . . . I didn't know you had a son," said Myra. I hadn't known either.

"Oh yiss," said Mrs. R. "But you don't neveh see him, 'cause he goes to voik at fife A.M. So he comes visit me foist." She patted my wife on the hand. "I vanted you should heff sump'n t' remember me mit," she said.

"They're just beautiful, Mrs. Rosenbaum," said my wife. "And it was so nice of you to want to give them to me. But I'd have remembered you anyway. I'll see you after the operation, and I'll bring you some more chicken soup."

Mrs. Rosenbaum just smiled at Myra. "I von't forget you, dear," she said.

The next morning, the surgeons had barely opened Mrs. Rosenbaum's abdomen when she suffered another heart attack, so they closed up the incision and sent her down to the morgue. Somebody suggested that she couldn't have been saved by anything short of a complete body transplant. I didn't argue.

10

The Dumping Syndrome

The Dumping Syndrome is a well-known medical entity. It occurs in people who have had their stomachs removed, usually because of intractable ulcer disease. The name derives from the tendency of food, in these patients, to cause intestinal hypermobility when it hits the small intestine without first having been altered in the customary fashion by gastric digestion. This hypermobility then causes the ingested food to be zipped down the pike—dumped, as it were—and in the process some impressive diarrhea is produced. Those who suffer from the condition don't speak of it in kindly terms.

At The Vue, all of us on the house staff suffered from a dumping syndrome, too. What was dumped on the Bellevue doctors was, to be specific, patients. To be even more specific, it was unwanted patients from other hospitals. As I've already mentioned, Bellevue Hospital was never allowed to refuse admission to a patient. Not for any reason. Thus any person who came to The Vue and was found to be in need of hospitalization was forthwith admitted. Though not a single intern or resident would have admitted it out loud, we viewed this policy as a source of pride. Frequently, though, we also considered it a source of severe irritation, and we weren't the least bit bashful about giving voice to that sentiment.

Our irritation arose from the fact that the staff at every other hospital in the city knew the way the game was played, and the rules were all in their favor. Private hospitals or municipal, it didn't matter. They were all aware that the gates of The Vue never swung shut, and that was all the ammunition they needed. It meant that any time they didn't wish to admit a particular patient, they had only to shove him or her into an ambulance and point the vehicle toward First Avenue and Twenty-sixth Street.

It was really just that easy. There was no necessity for fancy excuses, so that at least 95 percent of the transfer slips read simply, No Beds. The commotion that the average Bellevue intern produced upon receiving a patient from Puspocket General with a No Beds slip was truly impressive. He shrieked. He howled. He beseeched the Almighty to strike dead the miserable prevaricating camel driver who had perpetrated the heinous crime. At least once a week, an intern in this situation would dial Puspocket's administrative office, assume his sweetest manner, and say, "This is Admitting. Would you please give me the census on Male Medicine?" Then, when the administrator would tell him that Male Medicine was only 76 percent full, he'd identify himself, and in his most righteous and wounded tones, would demand to know why, in that case, they had seen fit to send a patient to The Vue with a No Beds slip. At that point, the administrator would apologize for the "error" and rapidly hang up, leaving the intern with nothing to do but splutter and then go and work up the patient who, of course, had already been officially admitted to Bellevue.

What manner of patient was it that caused such ghastly ructions to reverberate through the halls of The Vue? You may be certain that no municipal politician or television actress was ever dumped onto The Vue after having being told there were no beds at the hospital of his or her choice. However, most respectable institutions looked with general disfavor upon addicts and prostitutes, and an inordinate number of these individuals found themselves riding meat wagons on a one-way trip to the shore of the East River. Nor was there often room at the inns for ninety-year-old nursing home denizens who happened to contract pneumonia. And, of course, it goes without saying that persons deficient in both money and health insurance were provided very rapid motorized bums' rushes. Sometimes, the fact that a patient needed admission in the middle of the night constituted sufficient grounds for transfer: Why should a Puspocket doctor stay up all night when the Lord in His kindness and mercy hath provided Bellevue interns?

But there is some good in even the worst of things, and this was certainly true of the Bellevue dumping syndrome. It should be apparent from what has been said that a prime motivating factor behind many dumps was the laziness of the dumper. Hence, difficult cases were frequently stuffed into an ambulance and sent to The Vue; it was easier to do that than to try to figure out what was wrong with the patient. We received some of our most interesting cases in this fashion, and although routine dumps sent us into memorable tantrums, we never so much as whimpered when the meat wagon from Puspocket disgorged a fascinoma at our feet. At these times, in fact, our emotions ran close to downright gratitude.

Alberta Cowens was such a patient. She easily qualifies as the most spectacular dump I ever received.

The Cowens saga began for me on a January night shortly after I had begun a senior medical-student elective on obstetrics. The service was short one resident, so they decided to utilize me in that capacity. Giving me the title of sub-resident, they taught me the necessary skills and then plugged me into the vacant slot to help cover the labor and delivery suite. My sense of self-importance promptly assumed record proportions.

Fortunately for me and for the patients, my first week was a pretty quiet one, allowing me to concentrate fully on each woman as she came in and labored. As the second week began, the workload remained light, and about eight o'clock one evening I found myself totally patientless, a rare condition at The Vue. I sprawled on an unused stretcher and listened as the nurse told me stories about Jamaica, her native country. In the middle of the Kingston market, between the fruit venders and the hat weavers, the doors to the delivery suite swung open, crashed into the walls, and the aide from A.O. pushed in a stretcher with a black woman on it. She was holding her protuberant belly, and her facial expression indicated that there had been days when she had felt better. The aide handed me a slip of paper, which on inspection proved to be a transfer note. It read, "Premature Labor—No Beds." I sighed, and turned to examine the patient.

She was complaining of pains in her belly and was in her thirty-fourth week of pregnancy. It quickly became apparent, however, even to inexperienced me, that she was not having uterine contractions, so she could not be in labor. I proceeded to check her thoroughly from shoulder blades to pubis. I listened to the baby's heartbeat, which was perfectly normal, and I poked and jiggled all over her belly. As I moved the baby around, she told me that that made her pain worse. I said I was sorry, promised to be more gentle, and furrowed my forehead so as to look properly cogitative. Then I did a pelvic examination.

After I completed my maneuvers, Mrs. Cowens told me that she was thirty-five years old and that this was her third pregnancy. The trouble had started during her fourth month, when she had had an attack of severe abdominal pain, nausea, and vomiting. At the time she and her family had been living in Houston, and she had gone to the emergency room of a hospital in that city. There she had sat, doubled over, for an hour and a half, after which time she was shown to an examining cubicle. Here she waited for another forty-five minutes. Finally the doctor came in.

"He was young, and in a mighty big hurry," Mrs. Cowens recalled, and I felt my cheeks get warm. "Can't say I really blame him too much, though. The place was packed with bad-sick people; you know, shootings, and heart attacks, and stuff like that. He just read what the nurse wrote down on my paper, and said real fast that bellyaches and vomiting were normal for pregnant women. Then he started to leave."

Mrs. Cowens smiled and shook her head. "That kinda got me mad,".she said. "'Doctor,' I told him, 'I've had two babies already, and I *never* felt pains like this before. And by my fourth month, I was always finished vomiting. This pregnancy just doesn't feel right.'

"The doctor was almost out the door by then. He looked back over his shoulder and hollered that every pregnancy is different, and I shouldn't worry about it, and I oughta register for care in their clinic.

"Well, there wasn't much I could say to him since I was all by myself in the room then, so I got up and went on home. My husband was mighty angry, let me tell you; why, he was all set to take me right back there and *make* that doctor at least give me an examination. Or else he wanted to call up a private doctor, and that made me laugh. 'You know we don't have the money for that,' I told him. 'Let's just wait and see what happens. Maybe it really will get better.' Besides, we were going to move to New York less'n a month later, and I figured I could go see a doctor when we got here."

However, the job that was awaiting Mr. Cowens didn't work out for another three and a half months, so the family didn't move until Mrs. Cowens was almost eight months along. During this time her abdomen progressively enlarged, and the baby began to move—but not in the usual gentle, fluttery fashion. The movements seemed to her to be especially strong, and often were followed by knife-like pain under the ribs, bouts of cold sweat, and vomiting. But since the symptoms never persisted long, Mrs. Cowens did not again seek medical care in Houston. Upon her arrival in New York, she registered at a prenatal clinic and had an appointment there for the following week. However, a renewed attack of lower abdominal pain caused her once again to seek care on an emergency basis. Upon her arrival at the prenatal clinic, she said the doctor there had dismissed her with a glance as a routine case of premature labor, and she had been loaded into the meat wagon and shipped downtown to The Vue.

I told Mrs. Cowens that I thought nothing was seriously wrong. I further explained that her baby was lying transversely in her uterus, which I thought might be due to the fact that her cervix was displaced far forward, indicating that the uterus was tilted at an abnormal angle. Thus I supposed that the baby was wedged in unusually tightly, causing the fetal movements to be more painful than average. The nausea and vomiting I attributed to this same uterine trauma. It was really a beautiful explanation. However, as things turned out, it was completely untrue. Fortunately Mrs. Cowens remained satisfied that my intentions had been good, and never held my diagnostic disaster against me.

I suggested that Mrs. Cowens try to get an earlier clinic appointment at the other hospital, but she shook her head. "Don't want to go to them no more," she said firmly. "It's a little outa the way, but I want to come here and have my baby. It's the first place they ever gave me an examination and tried to tell me what's the matter. Fact is, I want you to be my doctor."

I promptly set a new record for head size. My conscience whispered that it might be proper, after all, to inform my petitioner of my true lowly status, but I silenced the nagging voice with the thought that if the Bellevue obstetrics department had seen fit to permit me to function as a doctor, then there was no reason why I should not do just that. So although the residents assigned to the delivery room did not customarily go to the Clinic, I told Mrs. Cowens that I'd be delighted to take on her case, and asked the nurse to arrange a clinic appointment for her the next afternoon.

When I arrived at the Clinic to see Mrs. Cowens, I passed Julian Armstrong, one of the senior residents. "I'm going to work up a lady I saw in labor and delivery last night," I said to him. "That's okay, isn't it?"

Julie grinned. "Sure, that's great," he said. "One less for us to do. Have a good time." As I walked away, he called after me, "If you want, holler when you're done, and I'll check her out for you."

I thanked him and went into the examining room, where Mrs. Cowens received me warmly. Her attack of pain had gone away shortly after she had left The Vue the night before, and had not returned. I reexamined her and found her physically unchanged from the previous examination. So I filled out her chart and went to look for Julie Armstrong.

Julie was busy. He walked quickly into the room, greeted the patient, and scanned the chart. Noticing my report of a transverse fetal lie, he perfunctorily felt the abdomen, and grunted in assent. "Don't forget to give 'er iron and vitamins," he said, as he charged out the door.

So, because he was in a hurry, my senior resident also failed to make the diagnosis, and I learned another valuable lesson: never trust anybody.

The remainder of Mrs. Cowens' pregnancy was relatively uneventful, although she did continue to suffer from periodic attacks of pain and gastrointestinal upsets. On a few occasions she was on the verge of calling the hospital, but the symptoms disappeared as suddenly and as mysteriously as they had arrived. She kept all her weekly appointments with me, at which times I gingerly examined her abdomen and assured her that the baby had not changed its manner of presentation. About three weeks before her due date, with the baby still lying transversely, I told her that there was only a slight chance that it would convert to a normal longitudinal lie, and that a caesarean section would be necessary to deliver the child safely. I made certain she understood that she was to report to the hospital immediately upon the onset of labor.

Six days later, Mrs. Cowens was wheeled into the labor and delivery area at The Vue. She told us she had been awakened from sleep by cramping pains in her abdomen, superimposed upon which were frequent, violent movements on the part of the baby. Doubled over, she had half-crawled, half-walked into the bathroom, and vomited explosively into the toilet. When she had finished, she walked carefully back to the bedroom, woke up her husband, and told him she thought they'd better go to the hospital. By the time they arrived, her pain had greatly intensified.

I examined Mrs. Cowens, and saw no reason to alter my original diagnosis. It merely seemed that she was in labor, and perhaps a bit on the nervous side. So I gave her an injection of Demerol and Phenergan to ease her pain and calm her down, and then called up the senior resident to tell him we had a transverse lie in labor who needed a caesarean section.

At that point Mrs. Cowens' luck took a turn for the good. My senior resident on call that evening was Vincent Ciccone. Vince was well known at The Vue as an intense worker and an extremely conscientious and knowledgeable doctor. His compulsive behavior was a perpetual source of exasperation to the rest of the residents, but we had to admit that it was also at times responsible for the successful outcome of a particularly difficult case. Most of the seniors would have told me to prepare the patient for surgery and then to call back when everything was ready. Vince came immediately to the labor suite.

When he arrived, he found Mrs. Cowens writhing on the examining table. He frowned as he touched her rigid abdomen, and she screamed in pain. His frown deepened as he did a pelvic examination and noticed the abnormally situated cervix. He made certain that she was not bleeding, and then, by checking her blood pressure, pulse, and general appearance, satisfied himself that she was not in shock. He listened to the loud, regular fetal heartbeat, and concluded that the baby was all right, at least for the moment. "But this isn't any ordinary transverse lie," he said tersely. "Get some blood for emergency cross-match, and then let's take her down to X-ray. Maybe that'll show us what's going on."

A half an hour later we were staring at an X-ray view box. Vince pointed toward the radiograph. "Look," he said. "The fetal spine is very poorly flexed, and the arms and legs aren't well folded at all. In fact, they're sticking out in all different directions. Give you any ideas?"

I shook my head.

"Okay, let's get a lateral view," said Vince.·

As we put the lateral film up onto the view box, Vince actually jumped up and down. "That just about clinches it," he hollered.

I stared at the film, utterly mystified. I couldn't even think of an intelligent question to ask.

"Look at the X-ray, Larry," snapped Vince. "The baby's bottom foot is overlapping the mother's spinal column.

"But that's impossible—if the baby's inside the uterus," I said slowly.

"Aha," Vince crowed. "And look here. There're all kinds of loops of intestine intermingled with the baby's body."

In his agitation, Vince almost shoved me back into the X-ray room. Mrs. Cowens was lying on the table on her side, clutching her abdomen, with her legs drawn up as far as her distended belly would allow. We helped her to turn onto her back, and then Vince gently inserted a thin metal probe through the cervix into the uterine cavity.

"Doesn't go terribly far at all," he said, giving me an affirmative nod.

The technician snapped a side view of Mrs. Cowens' abdomen. As the film came out of the developer, Vince grabbed it and thrust it up onto the viewing screen. He punched me firmly on the arm. "How does that grab you?" he shouted.

"I'll be damned," I mumbled. I couldn't stop gawking at the X-ray, which clearly showed the probe extending up into a uterine cavity whose small extent obviously could not contain a full-term pregnancy. Above and behind the probe, clearly separated from it, lay the fetus.

I finally turned around to look at Vince, but he wasn't there. He had gone across the room and was talking on the phone, gesticulating emphatically at the mouthpiece as he spoke. I walked toward him, and as I did, I heard him tell Dr. Allen Bean, our attending physician, to come right in and help him operate on a case of advanced abdominal pregnancy with a living fetus.

Most laymen are acquainted with the term ectopic pregnancy which they equate with a gestation in the fallopian tube. For the most part they're right, but all ectopic pregnancies are not tubal. Strictly speaking, an ectopic pregnancy is one which is located outside the uterine cavity. Aside from the tube, the pregnancy may be situated in the ovary, the uterine cervix, or the abdominal cavity. In most American localities, one out of every hundred to two hundred pregnancies is ectopic. Ovarian and cervical gestations account for only a tiny number of these, while the incidence of abdominal pregnancy is about 1:3500.

Quite understandably, throughout history, abdominal pregnancy has been a source of amazement and wonder to lay and medical observers. The Talmudic rabbis recorded the case of a child "which emerged from the abdominal side of the mother." Adherents to the Buddhist faith believe that their spiritual leader "was born through the right side or the armpit of his mother."

The first authentic recording of an abdominal gestation, however, is generally attributed to Albucasis, the famous Arabian physician who practiced in Cordova in Spain during the tenth century A.D. Albucasis described the case of a woman whose fetus had died undelivered, and who then conceived a second time. This fetus also died without being expelled. After an interval, an abscess appeared at the umbilicus which, upon rupture, exuded pus and two small bones. Astonished, the physician probed the abscessed cavity and extracted numerous bones, which he thought belonged to the two fetuses. The woman eventually recovered.

Many obstetrical historians believe that the first case of surgery for abdominal pregnancy with survival of both mother and baby was that of Elizabeth Nufer. The operation supposedly took place in Sigershausen, Switzerland, in the year 1500. The patient had appeared to be in labor with her first child for several days, but remained undelivered despite the attention of numerous midwives. Her husband, Jacob, the village swine gelder, finally decided that enough was enough, and took matters into his own hands. Assisted by two of the more courageous midwives, he "placed his wife upon a table and made an incision in her belly, just as he would have done in the swine. He opened the abdomen so neatly with one stroke of his knife that the child was extracted at once without harm." Both patients did amazingly well postoperatively.

Over the next four hundred years, European doctors performed and reported numerous operations for abdominal pregnancies, usually to remove retained dead fetuses, some of which had remained in place as long as forty-six years. Apparently, the first time a case of abdominal pregnancy came to surgery in the United States was in 1759, when John Bard operated on a certain Mrs. Stagg. The mother, but not the baby, survived.

With the passage of time, improved surgical techniques, the use of antibiotics, and matched blood transfusions have combined to lower the risk to the mother, though recently quoted modern maternal mortality figures of 6 to 15 percent are still high enough to inspire considerable anxiety in the mind of any obstetrician faced with such a patient.

The question arises as to the manner in which a pregnancy comes to develop in the abdominal cavity. Relatively few of these cases represent primary abdominal pregnancies, that is, where an egg, released from the ovary, falls into the abdominal cavity upon failure of the usually reliable tubal pickup mechanism. The felony is then compounded by a particularly enterprising spermatozoon, which traverses the entire length of the uterus and tube and passes into the abdomen, where it fertilizes the aberrant egg. The newly created embryo then does what comes naturally, sending its placental offshoots deep into the exterior of the uterus, the intestines, the bladder, the pelvic wall, or any other handy structure. In contrast, the majority of abdominal pregnancies are secondary, which means that they begin as the more common tubal type of gestation. Although most tubal pregnancies rupture, with massive and dramatic intra-abdominal hemorrhage, those destined to become abdominal pregnancies erode slowly through the wall of the tube, with little or no bleeding. Then, the placenta subsequently spreads out its attachments onto the surrounding pelvic structures while the fetus continues its development, essentially free in the abdominal cavity.

The exterior surface of the uterus, the intestines, and the peritoneal lining of the inner abdominal wall cannot supply nearly as hospitable an environment for the implanting and developing embryo as can the specialized uterine cavity. Therefore, in most cases of abdominal pregnancy, the abnormally situated placenta sooner or later reaches the limit of its impaired capacity to supply oxygen and nutrients to the fetus, which then dies. If this occurs early, the small fetus and placenta are broken down by the body's natural defenses, and the products are absorbed via the blood stream. However, if the fetus manages to reach a size too large to permit reabsorption, then some of the most amazing and unusual situations in medicine may ensue. The fetus may undergo desiccation and calcification, with formation of a lithopedion (literally, "stone man"). Some of these may be discovered many years later, at surgery, at autopsy, or when they block the birth canal during a subsequent labor. On other occasions, bacteria from the intestines may enter the dead fetus and cause formation of an abscess, which may then rupture through the abdominal wall (as in the case of Albucasis), or alternatively, into the bladder or rectum, with the ultimate passage of small bones by the urinary or the fecal route, a matter of much amazement and no little consternation to the passer and her physician. In probably no more than 5 percent of all abdominal pregnancies does the placenta eke out sufficient nutriment from its unlikely implantation site to support the growth of a fetus to viability.

Primarily because of its rarity, abdominal pregnancy often is not diagnosed until obvious signs of an intra-abdominal catastrophe force themselves upon the consciousness of the medical observer. From the beginning, Mrs. Cowens' symptoms were quite typical of the disease.

Very commonly, the first sign of trouble is a bout of abdominal pain during the second or third month, often accompanied by light vaginal bleeding. This probably is the time at which the pregnancy is eroding through the tubal wall and into the abdomen. From that point on, abdominal pain, nausea, and vomiting are frequent and severe, as the placenta burrows away at whichever organ happens to be available, and as the fetus grows and moves among the loops of intestines. As was the case with Mrs. Cowens, the fetus usually seems to be carried higher than is normal, and frequently it assumes a transverse orientation relative to the mother, rather than the normal vertical lie, with head down. Because of the displacement of the empty uterus by the growing pregnancy, the cervix may occupy an abnormal position in the vaginal canal: Mrs. Cowens' cervix was pushed forward, but depending on the location of the pregnancy, it might have been pushed backward or to the side. When this sign is recognized, sometimes the diagnosis can be made by feeling parts of the baby through the upper vaginal wall, next to the cervix, and therefore not within the uterus.

When abdominal pregnancy is thought probable, the diagnosis may be confirmed by the technique Vince Ciccone used. A metal probe placed within the uterine cavity will be seen on an X-ray to be adjacent to and separated from the fetus.

In point of fact, both Mrs. Cowens and her baby—but especially the baby—were fortunate that the doctor in the Houston emergency room was not more thorough and that I was not more experienced. Because of the very poor outlook for the baby, most obstetricians will operate to terminate an abdominal pregnancy as soon as the diagnosis has been made. To do otherwise is to run the risk that part of the placenta may separate from its attachments, producing massive, possibly fatal, hemorrhage. In addition, at surgery, unless the blood vessels supplying the placenta can be clearly identified and tied off, the placenta should be left in place after the baby has been removed. This will prevent the occurrence of heavy, unstoppable bleeding from the implantation site. In normal pregnancies, the post-delivery contraction of the uterine muscle fibers squeezes shut the huge blood vessels in the placental bed, preventing bleeding, but in abdominal gestation there is nothing to constrict the dilated arteries and veins after the placenta has been torn away from them. In contrast, when the abdominal placenta is left in place, it most often gradually reabsorbs, leaving just a small lump at the implantation site. Sometimes, however, the organ will become infected, producing an abscess. Or it may become painful, or even cause obstruction of the intestine. Any of these complications requires re-operation, but this is not as dangerous as the hemorrhage caused by separation of the placenta at the time of delivery of the child.

That was all I could think about as we wheeled Mrs. Cowens to the operating room. I wasn't altogether grateful to Vince Ciccone for making me aware of the potential disasters that could have been visited on our patient. By that time her belly was so tender we couldn't even touch it. I had made certain that the blood bank had six bottles of compatible blood ready to use and that they were getting even more ready. But now I knew that if there should be one wrong move at the operation, she would lose blood faster than we'd be able to run it in. I began to wish I had taken my elective in dermatology. Suddenly, it wasn't so much fun to be a sub-resident in obstetrics.

But there was no way out of it, so I took a deep breath and we wheeled her into the operating room. The anesthesiologist put her to sleep while Vince, Dr. Bean, and I scrubbed up. Then we put on our gowns. If any one had measured the adrenalin in my blood stream, I'd have probably made the Guinness Book of Records. Vince cut an incision between the pubic bone and the navel, and then opened the peritoneum, the membrane that lines the abdominal cavity. With that, huge quantities of amniotic fluid poured out over the patient, the table, the floor, and down our legs. What had happened was that the amniotic sac, or bag of waters, had broken while she had been home sleeping. This, then, explained her intense pain: amniotic fluid can be quite irritating to intra-abdominal tissues.

Vince then proceeded to open the peritoneum the length of the incision, and there was the baby, lying all tangled up in a mess of intestines. Grabbing the feet, he pulled the child out. It began to cry immediately, even before we had clamped and cut the cord. It was a little girl, and it appeared to be perfectly normal. We gave the baby to the pediatrician, and then looked to see what was left.

My first feeling was unmitigated relief: it was obvious that no blood was flowing. We cleaned out the rest of the amniotic fluid—very gingerly—and clamped the cord right next to the placenta.

That left us with quite a sight. Usually at surgery you can see the uterus, tubes, and ovaries, all lying in their appropriate places in the pelvis. But here I could only make out the right tube and ovary and the right half of the uterus. The whole left side of the pelvis was completely buried under the placenta. Just looking at it gave me the shivers. It was sitting on the top of the left side of the uterus, covering the tube and ovary, and extending over to the left wall of the pelvis, where it was solidly implanted over the left common iliac and hypogastric arteries. These vessels supply blood to the entire pelvis and lower left side of the body. Vince pointed out that the amount of blood that the placenta must have been tapping off them had to be absolutely staggering. "That's probably the reason the baby was able to survive all the way to term," he said. "The blood supply from these big arteries probably could have kept three kids going."

"What's your next step, Professor?" Dr. Bean asked Vince. "You want to go get that placenta?" I could see him grinning behind his mask.

"I don't even want to *look* too hard at the placenta," Vince answered. "All I want to do is close the belly quick and get the hell out of here."

Which is what he did. At the time, I shuddered as I thought of the postoperative complications she'd undoubtedly have, but remarkably, she didn't turn a hair. The next day, she was up and out of bed, and a week and a half later, she went home with the baby. Shortly thereafter, my time on the obstetrics service was up, but Vince kept me posted on her progress. He checked her at monthly intervals, and found that the placenta rapidly shrank down to become a little thickened area on the left side of the uterus. Mrs. Cowens complained periodically about a feeling of heaviness or fullness in her pelvis, but no more than that. And the baby did fine.

During one of these reports, I expressed regret and embarrassment at having so completely missed the diagnosis. Vince shook his head. "No reason for you to feel like that," he said. "Your mistake was one of inexperience, not of neglect. That's thoroughly excusable."

"I still wish I could have made the diagnosis," I said.

"Why?" Vince asked. "In the end, no harm was done to anyone. Matter of fact, you might look at it this way: if you had diagnosed abdominal pregnancy at thirty-four weeks, we'd have probably operated right then. And if we had, the baby might have died of prematurity. Those extra four weeks may have saved the baby's life."

"Wonderful," I said. "I did the right thing for the wrong reasons."

Vince laughed. "Somehow, I don't think Mrs. Cowens would argue the whys and the wherefores with you," he said. "The results are all she cares about." He paused for a moment. "Everything considered, this case has to be the luckiest dump in the history of The Vue."

11

A Receptacle for All Purposes

Of the seven body orifices that communicate with the outside world, only the mouth was designed to be used as an intake port. But man is nothing if not inventive, and he continues to try all possibilities. I've never heard of a dog or a cat that needed a Coke bottle extracted from its rectum; however, as described in a previous chapter, such operations have been performed in many hospital emergency rooms where humans are treated.

Since patients at Bellevue generally did run a bit to the bizarre, the foreign objects encountered in Bellevue orifices also were about as peculiar as one might imagine. Bellevue physicians were called upon to remove a fascinating assortment of material that had been lost in the different body openings. Every day we removed Q-tips from ears, wadded paper from nostrils, and a truly amazing variety of objects from rectums. Many of these were started on their travels up the wrong end of the intestinal tract as silly or drunken jokes. Others came to rest up there as the result of accidents during the sexual activities of homosexuals. Medical literature catalogs a large number of review papers which describe the odd things that the authors and/or their friends have removed from various rectums. The items range from bottles through bananas, hot dogs, knives, rubber hoses, and electric light bulbs. At least one of these bulbs was documented to still be functional upon its recovery. This was described with such pride that I wondered whether the author had offered his prize for display at the Smithsonian Institution. What a great ad that would have made for G.E. or Sylvania.

In most instances, the Bellevue Admitting Office doctors took care of these problems. However, there was one orifice which they never dared explore: the vagina.

109

Let a woman appear with a nasal, aural, or even a rectal bezoar, and she was promptly emptied and sent on her way. But let her even intimate that the offending substance had been secreted in her vagina, and with whitened countenance and quavering tones, the Admitting Office physician would cry, "Get her up to the gynecologist."

I have never been able to figure it out. Otherwise competent and considerate doctors invariably seemed to feel that it was necessary to awaken a certified womb-snatcher simply to effect removal of an object from a woman's vagina. You'd think they could at least have tried, but they never did. You may form your own conclusions regarding the matter. As an oft-awakened gynecology resident, I definitely had my own.

The majority of these referred cases were straightforward. For example, some of the patients were little girls. Large numbers of prepubertal females seem to regard the vagina as a first-class repository for appropriately shaped toys. Crayons, dolls' arms, chalk, and cotton balls all fit very nicely into a mini-crotch. What's more, the items are never discovered until they cause enough irritation to produce a discharge or some bleeding, at which time the mother brings the child in for evaluation. In point of fact, these foreign bodies can be anything but trifling. There was a recent report in a gynecologic journal relating the case of a grown woman with a very long history of severe, incapacitating pelvic infections who was finally demonstrated at surgery to have a bit of wire embedded beneath her vaginal wall. This wire was later identified as a part of a long-forgotten childhood toy. After its removal, the patient remained totally free of the symptoms which had troubled her for the preceding twenty-five years.

Another common problem involved removing a "missing Tampax." I never could understand how those things managed to get crammed way up into the very top of the vagina until one night after an unplanned and unscheduled nocturnal adventure when my wife called from the bathroom to request that I perform this bit of extirpative surgery on herself. Then, at last, I understood. With rare exceptions, the patients who had lost their tampons expressed surprise at how easily they were ultimately removed. Not just uneducated patients, either. Beatniks from Greenwich Village and college girls from the nearby Washington Square campus of N.Y.U. regularly expressed their gratitude and relief that a major abdominal operation would not, after all, be necessary. They invariably thought that the tampon had passed into the uterus, either remaining there or continuing along El Camino Real to become a free-lying foreign object in the abdominal cavity. Very few of them seemed to know that the connection between the vagina and the uterus is far too small to permit passage of a menstrual tampon. This, however, I could always understand. In that situation, my patients must have felt as I invariably do when my auto mechanic tries to get me to comprehend the nature of the malfunction of my car's engine.

But natually, life as the gynecology consultant to the Admitting Office was not all crayons and Tampax. As anywhere else in Bellevue, unusual patients abounded.

One such woman came timidly into the consultation room about 1 P.M. on a Sunday. Her A.O. slip identified her as Helen Jones, whose problem was "FB in Vag." (That's "foreign body in vagina.") The space provided for the referring doctor's history and physical examination were as untouched and pure as the West Virginny snow, and I quietly gnashed my teeth. Then, I asked Miss Jones what her FB was.

She was skinny and about thirty years old. Her pale face contrasted horribly with the red blotchiness around her nose and mouth. She wrung her hands and dripped a few tears onto her high-necked, sensible cotton-print dress. Then she let out a low moan and asked, "Do I have to tell you?"

I felt sorry for her. I really did. But I knew never to take a Bellevue patient's plea so seriously that I would end up with my own soft parts exposed. It was one thing to stick my neck out for a patient when I knew it was necessary for his or her care, but it was entirely a different matter to allow myself to be taken in by one of the excellent and experienced Bellevue con ladies. So I told Miss Jones that she did indeed have to tell me what had found its way into her vagina.

She wrung her hands again. "Why do I have to tell you?" she whispered.

"Because maybe you don't know what kinds of things I've removed from women here," I answered. "I've taken out knives and pieces of glass. One lady even had a small mousetrap."

"Oh, dear," she moaned. "It's nothing like that. It's nothing that can hurt you. Honestly it can't."

"I'm sorry," I said. "I can't take it out unless you tell me what it is. I really can't see why you can't tell me."

"I'm just too embarrassed." She began to weep again, and the blotches began to spread.

"Look, why don't you just tell me and we'll be done with it? I'm eventually going to see it anyway."

"I just can't. But I've got to have it out."

I asked the nurse to leave for a minute. Then I turned back to my nearly hysterical patient. "Okay, now there's no one here," I said. "Tell me what it is, and then I'll be able to go get it out. I won't even put it in your record. All right?"

No answer.

"Take a deep breath and let it out."

Miss Jones inhaled and then roared, "It was a . . . a . . ."

I leaned forward.

". . . lipstick," she exhaled in a hoarse whisper.

A lipstick! I sat back. What a letdown. But how in the hell had a lipstick gotten into her vagina?

I called the nurse in, and we got Miss Jones up onto the examining table. I thought there would be no problem. I picked up a speculum and tried to insert it. It would have passed more easily through a brick wall.

I took a closer look. It became apparent that whenever my finger contacted her vulva, she would tighten her muscles and convert her carefully preserved maidenhood into a truly sturdy fortress.

A wave of sadness passed over me. Poor Miss Jones. I pictured her lying alone as usual in her bed the night before, and wondering as she often did what it felt like. She probably reached for the lipstick on an impulse; it looked small enough. Then, after a while, it must have gotten a little slippery down there. Woops—dropped it in. Oh my God. I DROPPED IT IN!

I could picture Miss Jones's night of frantic, futile efforts at removal and the courage it must have taken for her to come in. I stopped poking around and quickly assured her that I'd leave her anatomically as she had always been. Then I gave her an intravenous dose of a tranquilizer. It didn't help very much. Now I could slip one finger into her vagina, barely far enough to just touch the lipstick, but no more than that. And when I tried to snare it with a surgical clamp, it kept slipping away.

I was almost ready to resort to anesthesia when I suddenly had another idea. I inserted my left index finger into her rectum and used it to stabilize the elusive cosmetic. Then it was fairly easy to clamp it via the vagina and, by a combined maneuver, to work it forward and out.

Despite my request that she stay until the tranquilizer had worn off, Miss Jones was on her feet as soon as I'd finished. She hastily weaved out the door, hoisting her panties as she went. By the time I realized she had left the lipstick behind, she was well out of sight. The nurse assured me that we had no need for it either.

Another patient I'll long remember represented a slight variation on the preceding theme. She was not an A.O. referral, but had come into the hospital to have a hysterectomy. She was a tall, thin Negro woman whose slender build accentuated the bulge in her lower abdomen that was caused by the huge fibroid tumors in her uterus. She was a delightful lady who gave funny and salty answers to most of the questions I put to her. When she laughed at her own jokes, her mouth looked like the Lost Nugget Mine. By her admission, she was the proprietress of one of the most popular—and definitely the cleanest—whorehouses in Harlem. "Y' be s'prised, Doctuh," she said. "We got lotsa white boys come up. We ain't prejidiced." She slipped me a sly smile.

"Come on now," I said. "I bet you put the white boys in the back of the house."

She burst into peals of laughter, and her teeth flashed brilliantly. "Gawd damn, you a funny li'l doctuh. You come by my place, I take good care o' you." Then she put on a mock serious expression, leaned forward, and stage-whispered, "Or you got one o' them wifes whut doan wan' their men messin' wif cullid wimmin?" This accompanied by the sly smile.

I assured her that my wife was not racially prejudiced but that she probably would take a dim view of my messin' wif any wimmin', cullid or otherwise. The patient laughed with gusto again.

By this time I was really enjoying myself. I asked her why she had come all the way down from Harlem to Bellevue Hospital. "OOOOOOH, Doctuh!" she said, opening her eyes so that she looked rather like Louis Armstrong. "Doan you know?" I assured her I didn't, but that she now had me more curious than ever.

"Waaaaal, it's like this. D' doctuhs at Hahlum Hosp't'l, dey fum C'lumbia. Dey use' t' treatin' dem rich 'n' faymis folks up by Harkness P'vilyun. So when it's dehr turn t' come spend a few mumfs at Hahlum, dey figguhs it's nuff fo' d' pore nigguhs jus' t'

have d' white doctuhs fum C'lumbia takin' care ov 'um. An' I tell y',
dey shore treats them pore nigguhs like pore nigguhs. But dat ain't
fer me, no sir. Ever'one in Hahlum knows, d' doctuhs at Bellevue
treet y' d' same no mattuh what culluh y' is. Why dey even treets d'
junkies nice, most times."

I didn't know whether or not she was putting me on, so I said
something to the effect that the Columbia doctors I knew seemed
like pretty nice guys. She stopped smiling and pointed her right
index finger at me, jabbing as she spoke; "Now, you a nice doctuh,
doan try gimme no sheet. Why d' hell ain't *yew* at Hahlum, huh?
No doctuh dere never talk t' me like yew do. Dey too damn good
to' joke aroun' a li'l wif an ol' nigguh whoremarm. Now, with
emphasis via the finger, "I'm tellin' you d' troof, so I doan wan' you
t' try 'n' sheet me, heah?"

I nodded, and she began to smile again. I decided it was time
for a change of subject, so I asked her whether she used drugs. I
quickly explained that if she did and I didn't know it, she might
have a fatal bout of cold turkey after her operation.

"Noooo-suh," she answered. "Nonna dat stuff fer me. An' y'
know whut else—I doan 'low dat crap in my place, neider. Dat's
why d' cops nevuh busts me."

"Is that the only reason the cops don't bust you?" I grinned.

"Well, I does pay a li'l bustin' 'surance too. But lotsa folks pay
dat, 'n' d' cops busts 'em ennyway. I know dem cops, dey jes' doan
like dat stuff 'n' dey doan like d' folks as uses it."

I smiled and told her it was time to do a pelvic examination.
The nurse put her up on the table. When I inserted the speculum
and looked around inside, I noticed that on the left side of her
vagina there was a nasty-looking green area surrounded by a gray
exudate. I poked at it with a probe, and frantically tried to
remember which vaginal infection might look like that. Then I
noticed that it was coming away on the probe, so I took out the
speculum and investigated with my gloved fingers. I pulled it all
out. It was a gray, papery, soggy mess. As I looked closer, I noticed
there was a number 10 on it. So I unfolded it and discovered that
her infection was a soggy, cruddy, but very legal ten-dollar bill.

"Hey," I shouted as I waved it in front of my patient's eyes.
"Look what I found."

She peered up from her supine position and her eyes lit up.
"Gawd *damn*, doctuh! I bin lookin' fer dat fer d' pas' fo' mumfs. I
fergot where I put it."

All of us—nurse, patient, and doctor—laughed until we were weak. Then I finished the examination. Unlike Miss Jones, this lady didn't leave her removed foreign body behind. After I had finished examining her, I washed the money off, dried it on a paper towel, and gave it to her. As she took it, I asked her to please put it in her bra this time. She slapped her thigh, flashed her golden smile, and collapsed in laughter again. "Gawd *damn*," she wheezed. "Betcha I'm the onlies' lady evuh went to a doctuh fer a op'ration 'n' made ten bucks on d' deal."

Without much doubt, the most dramatic case in this group was that of the woman who requested removal of a lost pickle fork. Yes, that's what I said. This patient appeared for consultation at 6 A.M. on a Sunday, and I was not in the best possible humor when I came down after having been awakened. Neither did my mood brighten when I saw her otherwise blank "FB in Vag" A.O. slip, but when she told me what the FB was, I immediately began to perk up. Who could be cranky when faced with a case demonstrating such originality, such flair, such *elan*? My curiosity became overwhelming. I told the patient that I would indeed check her out, and that she didn't *have* to elaborate, but if she wanted to tell me, I'd certainly love to know how a pickle fork had found its way into (or among?) her private parts. I wondered whether she had been trying to retrieve a previously lost pickle.

My tact proved to be unnecessary. She said that she didn't in the least mind telling me. "We were at a party, my boyfriend and me," she said. "About 'n hour ago, he says t' me, 'I think I'll have some breakfast', so he takes this pickle fork and rams it up my . . . uh . . ."

"Up your other end?"

"Yeah, up my other end." She snickered at me, and went on. "Well, he lets go of the fork, and then we can't find it. So we figure I better come in and have you guys check me out."

I assured her that this was indeed a fine idea, and then I asked her whether her boyfriend was with her.

She shook her head. "Oh, no. He was afraid you'd call the cops and have him arrested for assault or something."

Of course I'd have had no intention of calling the cops. I just thought it might have been interesting to meet this guy. Preferably from a good, safe distance.

In any case, we put her up on the table and I looked inside.

Nothing. I didn't see a single pickle fork. Then I inserted my fingers (gingerly) and examined her entire vagina. It was clean as a whistle. So I told the woman that the fork must have dropped out onto the floor without their having seen it.

"Oh, no," she said. "We checked all around, on the whole bed."

At this point I decided she was probably a drunk or just a practical jokester. "Well," I said. "There isn't anything in there. I've checked you thoroughly . . ."

"You sure did."

"Yes. And there just isn't a thing there."

"Okay." She thought for a minute and then shook her head. "Thanks anyway. Sorry I bothered you for nothing."

I told her it was all right and then went out of the examining cubicle while she got dressed. I sat down at the desk and began to write up the chart. At this point, the senior resident wandered in. He greeted me and asked me what I had been up to. I told him the story of the phantom pickle fork and grinned at him. He didn't grin back. "What'd the X-ray show?" he asked.

"X-ray! Why in hell would I get an X-ray?"

"Look, buddy," he said. "You're a first-year resident. By the time you're a wise senior resident like me, you won't ask why you get an abdominal X-ray when a Bellevue lady tells you there's a pickle fork in her vagina and you can't find it." He drummed his fingers on the desk.

I shrugged and went back into the examining room to tell the woman that the boss doctor thought we ought to get an X-ray, just to be safe. She was willing. A short while later, when her picture was developed, there indeed was the pickle fork, lying in her abdominal cavity, nestled snugly between a couple of loops of bowel. I cringed and called back my senior. He put his arm around me and asked whether I had learned something.

"Yes," I muttered. "But would you kindly tell me how you knew?"

"We all learn from our own experiences," he said. "More than once, when I was a first-year resident, I was lucky enough to have a sharp senior resident around."

We put the lady back on the examining table and searched around the top of her vagina for the puncture site through which the offending instrument would have had to pass, but we never found it. My senior resident explained that these punctures could be very small and bloodless, and often would heal amazingly quickly.

Because of the danger that the fork might eventually puncture the intestine and cause peritonitis, we took our patient directly to surgery. She turned out to be lucky. The fork lay free and was easily removed, and her intestinal tract was intact. The anesthetist leaned over and looked. When he saw the fork, he whistled.

"Man, that's mean-looking," he said. "What're you gonna do with it?"

"We won't give it back to the patient," said my senior resident. "When she finds her boyfriend, I'm afraid I know what she'll do with it."

The anesthetist looked back at his operative record sheet. "Hey," he yelled. "What the hell should I call this operation, anyway?"

The senior resident didn't hesitate a moment. "Why obviously," he said, "it's an exploratory laparotomy and a pickle-forkectomy—what else?"

All the singular Bellevue cases involving vaginas did not have to do with foreign objects. At The Vue, even the natural vaginal contents sometimes became aberrations.

For example, a woman was sent for gynecological evaluation because she was complaining of unusual vaginal bleeding. I came in to find her ready for examination, and moaning and weeping hysterically. She was Puerto Rican and spoke no English. The referral slip said she was twenty-three years old, although she looked ten years older than that. I asked whether she were in pain; she shook her head no. When I looked into her vagina, I thought the blood there was similar in appearance to that found with a normal menstrual period. When I asked her in which way this bleeding was different from her normal menstrual flow, she just shrugged.

At this point, in the face of her hysteria, I decided my Spanish was betraying me. So I called for a female Puerto Rican nurses' aide and told her to ask the patient exactly what was the matter. I left the room so as not to inhibit the conversation.

About twenty minutes later, the aide came out. "You ain't gonna believe this, Dr. Karp," she said.

I told her I'd believe anything.

"Well, sir, this lady, she got her first baby when she was thirteen years old. Then she had a baby every year—eleven of them now—and this is the first time she ever had a period.

"You're right, after all," I said. "I don't believe it."

"No, really, Dr. Karp. I checked it out. She had her first baby before she ever had a period, and she always got pregnant right away afterwards."

"Jesus Christ," I muttered. "What are we going to do with her?"

"Oh, don't worry, Dr. Karp. I told her about periods, that they come when you're not pregnant, and it's normal, and all that stuff. Then I gave her a Kotex and told her to go ask her grandmother—she lives with her—and then I gave her a clinic appointment so you guys can give her some pills or tie her tubes or something."

My very favorite vaginal story began one night at 2 A.M. with a frantic phone call from the examining room. "Dr. Karp, you on GYN call?" asked the night nurse. "Come quick, we got a lady hemorrhaging."

I pulled on my pants and tied my shoes as I ran down the two flights of stairs. Arriving at the gynecology examining suite, I hurriedly asked where the patient was. The nurse pointed to a room, and I ran in. Introducing myself perfunctorily, I spread the patient's legs, put in a speculum, and looked. There was no blood at all.

I looked again. Then I shook my head and moved the speculum around. Still no blood. I pulled out the speculum and put my fingers in. All her organs seemed normal, and on removing my fingers, there was no blood at all on them. I began to get sore.

"Hey," I said to the patient, "I thought you were hemorrhaging. I don't see any blood at all."

The woman sat up. She was about fifty years old and weighed two hundred pounds, with a fat red face topped off by a disarrayed mess of white Brillo. I don't think I've ever seen anyone else so irate.

"You must all be nuts here," she yelled. "I've never seen such a bunch of crazy people."

"What the hell . . ."

"Shut up. I'm talking. I come in and say I'm bleeding to death and some loony nurse rips off my pants and puts me up on a table. Then some jerky young punk of a doctor sticks things up my crotch. What the hell does all this have to do with a nosebleed?" As if for emphasis, bright red blood began to spurt from her left nostril, and she jabbed at it with a bloodstained handkerchief.

The nurses' aide burst into uncontrollable giggling. I'm sure I looked as though I had been poleaxed. I checked the A.O. referral slip. It bore one word: "Hemorrhaging." I quickly apologized to the patient, showed her the slip, and explained the misunderstanding. Then I told her that if she would get dressed, I'd take her back to Admitting, and get her nosebleed seen to by the Ear, Nose, and Throat specialist. She looked at me dubiously.

We went downstairs, entered the A.O. by the back door, and I ensconced the lady in an examining room. Then I ran up to the nurse in charge and breathlessly cried, "Get ENT quick: there's a lady in the back room hemorrhaging from her nose.

The nurse fumblingly managed to get the call through, and I slipped back to the examining room. I stayed with the patient for a few minutes until I heard the voice of the nurse out front: "She's in back, Doctor, hurry; she's hemorrhaging." I gave the patient a grin and a salute, both of which she returned.

"Goddamned craziest place I ever saw," she muttered, as I eased out the back door.

12

You Rape 'Em, We Scrape 'Em

The other night my wife looked up from the paper to ask me whether I knew that until the child-labor laws were passed, it was routine for children to work fourteen-hour days in factories. "It even says," she added, "that when the reformers first tried to get Congress to pass the laws, most of the places told them it was none of their business, that it was a 'local problem.'" She looked at me in righteous indignation.

I think that my wife's disbelief over the horrors of child-labor abuses will be as nothing compared to the reaction of the average twenty-first century American as he contemplates the hideous abortion-related statutes that his forebears have had to live through and with. The American of the future may find it incredible that, at one time, a woman was forced to bear a child she did not want, perhaps one that was destined to be born devastatingly and incurably ill. It may be difficult for our great-grandchildren to imagine the dreadful diseases that their ancestors contracted in desperate attempts to end unwanted pregnancies.

It was only during the late 1960's that a few states began to relax some of their ultra-restrictive abortion laws, but the major change came in 1973, when the United States Supreme Court ruled that termination of a pregnancy before the seventh month should properly be a matter for private decision by a woman and her physician. This in effect created abortion on request, which in turn brought forth its own associated set of new problems. However, these have been minor in comparison to what went before and, by and large, the law seems to be working well. For instance, last year in New York, not a single maternal death was caused by an illegal abortion. That in itself is a miracle. While I was working at

Bellevue, the gynecology ward usually held one or two women whose kidneys and livers had been destroyed by the poisons produced by the bacteria which had been introduced into their reproductive tracts via the filthy instruments of their abortionists. The private hospitals in the city made haste to ship these women to us. Most of them would live for a week or two, and then die of kidney or liver failure. All we could do was to try to keep them and their families as comfortable as possible.

Of course, all the patients who underwent illegal abortion didn't die. In fact, most criminal abortions proceeded without incident. They'd have had to. Otherwise, since approximately a million illegal abortions were being performed each year, the entire female population of the United States might have been wiped out in fairly short order. During my residency, each day would bring six or ten bleeding women to Bellevue, where we would empty their uteri of residual tissue by dilatation and curettage (or dusting and cleaning, as one patient put it). Then, the next day, the patients would go home, little the worse for wear. Many would be back soon, though. And repeatedly.

Of necessity, any high-volume business runs heavily to the routine, and a good deal of this work was repetitious and not terribly interesting. But Bellevue being Bellevue, what potential existed for variation was expressed to the fullest degree.

One of the residents who trained at The Vue a few years before my time was Dr. Ralph Wynn. Dr. Wynn is presently chairman of the department of obstetrics and gynecology at Abraham Lincoln Medical School in Chicago, and is an internationally known figure in medical education circles. Dr. Wynn's field of special expertise is the placenta. I once heard him deliver a lecture on the subject, during which he described the episode which had originally triggered his fascination for afterbirths. It seems that one night, when he was a first-year resident, an individual from the parade of incomplete abortions that passed under his care presented him with a chunk of tissue she said she had passed. Being a thorough man, Dr. Wynn examined her, and being a logical man, he was perplexed by the fact that her physical findings indicated the presence of an intact, healthy, early pregnancy. So, being a brilliant man, Dr. Wynn then put a slice of the tissue under his microscope, and with the help of some comparative anatomy textbooks, determined that the tissue was in fact cat placenta. When confronted with the findings, the patient confessed that she had saved the placenta from her cat's litter earlier that day and had brought it to the hospital in the hope that she'd be able to trick a doctor into emptying her uterus by curettage. By such quirks is the course of history changed. Had someone other than Dr. Wynn been on duty that night, the chances are very good that the lady would have succeeded in her plan. She'd have had her abortion, and a great deal of valuable research on the structure and function of the human placenta might never have been done. Dr. Wynn didn't say what he had done with the patient after she had confessed. I think he should have aborted her. An original and imaginative effort like that should not have gone unrewarded.

One particular patient that I treated for an incomplete abortion was a Negro woman in her mid-thirties who immediately impressed me as being an unusually cool customer. She sauntered into the GYN examining area, sat down opposite me, and smiled. Her self-assurance took me aback. The usual patient in her condition was wheeled or rolled in, screeching bloody murder. This woman, however, presumably in midabortion, promptly made herself at home, and calmly wished me good evening. I began to record her history; she had the usual story of cramps and bleeding during the past several hours. Then I asked her how many children she had had.

"Three," she answered.

"And have you ever lost a pregnancy before?" I asked her.

"Oh, yes." She smiled pleasantly. "This is my twentieth."

I dropped my pen on the desk and stared at her. I was certain that I was in the presence of the world's champion aborter. Either that or she was trying to fudge her way into the Guinness Book of Records. "How in the devil have you managed to have twenty miscarriages?" I asked.

"No trouble," she smiled. "This is the first one I've ever had to come to the hospital for."

I smiled smugly. Now I understood. Many women believe that if a menstrual period happens to come a few days late, this represents an early abortion (they may be right, by the way). Since very few women are perfectly regular in their menstrual patterns, I figured that I had just happened to get a compulsive calendar counter. I stopped talking to myself long enough to ask her what seemed different this time that had brought her to the hospital.

"Well, I just couldn't get it all out."

The hounds of uncertainty began to gnaw at my hocks. "You couldn't get all what out?" I asked her.

Now it was her turn to look uncertain. "You *are* a female doctor, aren't you?" she asked.

I assured her that I was indeed a gynecologist.

"Well, then you ought to know what I mean. I couldn't get all of the baby and afterbirth out."

At this point I decided to raise the white flag. I flashed what I hoped was a nice, confidence-inspiring smile, and asked her just how she had tried to get all the baby and the afterbirth out.

"Well, Doctor," she said. "I used a rat-tail comb. I just stick it up inside there and swish it around and, in a little while, the whole thing comes out, just as neat as you please. But this time I kept on bleeding and having cramps, so I figured there must still be a piece up there."

"Now come on," I said. "Do you really expect me to believe that?"

The woman got up from her chair. I thought I had made her angry and that she was going to leave, but she walked into an examining cubicle. As she pulled the curtain, she smiled back at me, and said, "Just a minute, and I'll show you. You can see for yourself how it works."

A few minutes later, she bid me enter. A nurse that I had hastily rounded up went in with me. There was the patient, squatting on the floor. Between her feet she had a little round mirror on a stand, focused upward so it gave her a beautiful view of her cervix. From her pocketbook she produced a rat-tail comb and, referring to the image in her mirror, she deftly inserted the rat-tail into her uterus, gave it a couple of lighthearted twirls, and zipped it out. "Okay?" she said, with a faint but definitely observable note of triumph in her voice.

I felt dizzy. Using sterile instruments with the greatest caution, physicians sometimes perforate uteri while performing therapeutic abortions. Yet here was this crazy lady who had done twenty successful procedures on herself with a rat-tail comb, suffering as a complication only one piece of retained placenta. For this, my mother had had to send me to medical school. I lamely asked the lady how she had managed to devise her ingenious technique.

She straightened up. "Oh, I learned it from my momma. She said she must have used it on herself about fifty times. Never missed, either," she said, and grinned at me. "Momma always said she was gonna use it when she was pregnant with me, but she changed her mind at the last minute. Bet she was sorry sometimes, too."

I let that go by. "If you've got all the kids you want," I asked her, "why don't you get your tubes tied?"

Her eyes widened and she said, "My goodness, Doctor, I'm scared silly of having an operation."

My knees weakened a bit more.

"Besides," she added, "that might make me lose my nature. And I wouldn't like that, not one bit."

It always does my heart good to witness progress in medicine. A new technique is developed and perfected, and then it filters into general medical practice. This evolutionary process may be illustrated by the case of a young Bellevue miss who appeared one evening with an imminent miscarriage at almost the midpoint of her pregnancy. Aside from the fact that there was no way to save the baby, all was well, and the girl herself was in no danger. It was her first pregnancy, and I tried to console her by suggesting that probably things would go better next time. She smiled a little patronizingly at me, and explained that she hadn't wanted the baby and had had the abortion induced.

I was taken aback at that, and muttered, "Oh, good." But then it occurred to me that abortions were very difficult to perform and therefore to obtain halfway through pregnancy. So I asked her how she had done it.

She took a deep breath. "Well," she said, "me an' my boyfriend—he paid for the abortion—we went to this ol' lady's house. She does abortions, y' know."

I nodded my head. I knew. Or at least I thought I did. The girl drew in a fresh supply of air and went on. "Well, the ol' lady said I wuz too far along fer her to put something up me, so she wuz gonna do whut the doctors do. So she put a teaspoon a salt from the table inna glass a water—I tell y', Doc, I thought she wuz nuts—then she poured it all inna big hypodermic needle," (she meant syringe) "an' then she injected it all inna my belly." For proof, the girl triumphantly showed me the little needle mark on her lower abdomen. "Then, when we left, she said when the pains started, I should come to the hospital. So," she beamed up at me, "here I am."

"How much did it cost you?" I whispered.

"Two hundred bucks."

For a minute I just stood there, quietly jibbering. In 1965, intrauterine injections of salt solutions were just beginning to achieve medical acceptance as a means of terminating pregnancies too far advanced to permit safe dilatation and curettage. Doctors carefully measured out quantities of salt water not considered to be excessive, and with the greatest care and stringent precautions, injected the solutions into pregnant uteri. The reason for the ultra-careful behavior lay in the fact that the infusions had lethal potentialities if the salt were to reach the blood stream too rapidly or if infection happened to be introduced into the uterus. There were also a number of other non-lethal, but still serious, complications. And here, some old woman had scooped salt off her kitchen table and shot it right in—I just couldn't stand it. "Who was the woman—what was her name?" I barked.

The girl gave me a no-no motion of her index finger. "Hain't gonna tell yuh that," she smirked. "You must think I'm pret-ty dumb."

I was too mad to tell her that I thought in fact that by comparison and for many reasons, she made cretins look like Einsteins. I explained to the girl that although she had come through all right, it was terribly dangerous to inject unsterile salt water willy-nilly into someone's uterus. I also told her that in no way would she herself be persecuted or prosecuted, but that I was only interested in preventing another girl from being mutilated or killed. No dice. All I got was, "Hain't gonna tell yuh, so yuh might ez well quit askin'." So finally I quit askin'.

Very likely, until the 1973 Supreme Court decision, that old midwife somewhere in the wilds of Brooklyn was still pulling in a quick couple of hundred now and then by salting out an occasional baby. The perceptive reader will at once recognize the nature of the evils related to unrestricted abortion statutes: for example, augmentation of the welfare rolls.

The Bellevue clientele utilized an endless variety of techniques in their attempts at abortion. One night, the hospital attendants raced up a three-hundred-or-so-pound woman to GYN. She was screaming like a fire siren: her wail of "Ooooooooooooooooooooooooooooooh" started low in the bass range, ended in mezzo-soprano, and finally was punctuated with a highly emphatic "Lawd!" Over and over. The nurses quickly stripped her and put her up for examination. One nurse ran out and called me, "Better get in fast,

Dr. Karp. She's got a positive Thom McAn sign." This meant that the patient's shoes and feet were covered with blood, thereby indicating the presence of brisk vaginal bleeding. So I trotted into the examining room and introduced myself. As I put in a speculum, a gigantic clot came through it and hit the floor. Now *I* had a positive Thom McAn sign. Then, when I tried to put the speculum back, the lady clamped her enormous thighs together and started her siren going again.

I quickly decided that I was not going to be of much use with my right hand pinned in the patient's crotch while her continuing hemorrhage trickled down my sleeve into my armpit. So I requested that the lady cease and desist from her vise-like behavior.

"Oooooooooooooooo-oh, Doctor—you'se gonna hurt me."

I assured the woman that I would employ the utmost gentleness and that were she not to release my arm forthwith (a) she would bleed to death, and (b) my hand would fall off. She relaxed.

To the rising and falling of the siren's wails, I once again tried to begin my examination. And once again a tremendous quantity of blood hit the floor, and the walls began to close in on me from both sides. I gently reminded the patient that that was a no-no, and she managed to relax again. Finally, I was able to spot the source of the bleeding. I was surprised to see it was not coming from the uterus, but from an actively spurting blood vessel at the base of a large crater at the edge of the urethra (the external opening of the urinary system). I walked up to the head of the table and asked my refugee from the Hook and Ladder Brigade what she had put into her vagina.

"Got me some purple pills fum a lady," she gasped. "Tol' me to put 'em way inside, in a li'l hole I'd feel." With that, the patient leaned over the edge of the examining table and vomited on my Thom McAns.

Such was my first professional exposure to potassium permanganate, a chemical that was used fairly often in abortion attempts. Women inserted it into their vaginas, where its corrosive effect produced heavy bleeding. Some of the patients really did believe that the vaginal hemorrhage would eventuate in miscarriage. The better-informed women did it in an attempt to trick a neophyte physician into performing an abortion. They tried to make him believe that the vaginal bleeding was really of uterine origin, and that the doctor would only be completing a miscarriage already begun and fated to continue.

In any event, my patient was going into shock from blood loss, so we gave her a transfusion, and zipped her up to the operating room, where we could repair the damage under anesthesia. The woman had severely injured her urethral opening, and we feared for her eventual urinary function, but somebody somewhere liked her, and when her catheter was removed a couple of weeks later, her urine passed strictly on schedule.

During her stay on the ward, I got to know her pretty well. She told me about her seven other children at home, and how difficult it was to take proper care of them on welfare payments, but how she kept forgettin' to take that li'l pill at the wrooooong time. I assured her that we'd tie her tubes at the termination of her current pregnancy.

Naturally, Dr. Karp was on duty the night she returned, seven months later, to deliver her lovely nine-pound girl. A week after this event, as she prepared to leave the hospital, babe in arms and fallopian tubes in formaldehyde, she flashed me her mile-wide grin and thanked me for my contribution to her care. I told her she was welcome. "Doctor Karp," she said, "since you wuz so nice to me all 'long, I want you to help me name mah li'l gal. I'm plum outta names." She giggled.

I stifled the urge to tell her that I thought Permanganate would be elegant, lovely, and thoroughly appropriate. We settled on Christine.

One Friday afternoon, while I was sitting in the GYN emergency room, I realized that it was quiet: we hadn't seen a single patient for at least three hours. This was usually a portent of imminent disaster, and when the messenger from the Admitting Office brought in a frail, nervous-looking little lady, I began to get bad vibes. In a few minutes the nurse told me that the patient was ready, so I went in to examine her.

She may have been the most unattractive woman I have ever laid eyes on. The note from admitting said she was thirty-one, but she looked much older. Her hair had apparently started out the day drawn back in a bun; now it was flying all around her head and face, Medusa-style. A combination of acne and blotchy flushing contrasted with the chalky pallor of the rest of her skin. Her eyes looked glazed, and she was shaking all over. I asked her what was wrong. Something was, obviously.

"I'm having a miscarriage," she whimpered.

I checked her temperature. It was over 102°. "Did you do anything to bring it on?" I asked.

At that point the white parts of the lady's face turned even whiter. "Are you going to—you won't—call—you won't tell—the police?" she stammered. She was shaking so hard from both chills and fear that she dropped her little black pocketbook onto the floor; she pounced on it and clutched it again to her bosom.

I assured her I had no intention of calling the police, but that I simply wanted to know because some techniques of self-induced abortion are particularly hazardous and necessitate special treatment or special precautions.

She began to cry and then started to moan, "I did it. I did it. Oh, Lord, I did it. Will you treat me anyway?"

I told her I would, and asked her how she had done it. She sighed deeply and brushed the snakes to the back of her head. "I'm a . . . a social worker," she said. "From Indiana. I tried to have an abortion back home, but . . . but no one would do it. Then my supervisor found out I was pregnant, and I got fired from my job." She dabbed at her eyes and went on. "She said I wasn't any . . . any better than . . . our clients."

"So I took all my money and decided to come to New York. I thought I could certainly get an abortion here. But I was in the city three whole days and I couldn't get a single doctor to do it. I offered them every cent I had—every single penny—but not one of them would help me." The pitch of her voice hit the hysterical level, and she shrieked on, "Every cent I own I offered, and it didn't do any good. Look! Look! I'll show you." With this, she flung her little pocketbook open and money burst out. Bills flew around the room. Tens and twenties fluttered to the floor. A hundred settled on top of the speculum on the table. "Twelve hundred dollars," she screamed, "and no doctor would touch me for less than two thousand."

I helped her pick up the money and put it back into her purse. Twelve hundred dollars—three months' salary! I felt absolutely giddy. I wondered what I'd have done if I had lived in Hadleyburg at the time when Mark Twain's stranger was passing through.

The social worker from Indiana calmed down a bit at that point, and went on with her story. "When I couldn't find a doctor to help me, I finally got desperate. Last night, I was in my room at the Y and I just couldn't stand it anymore. So I . . . I took a . . . coat hanger, and dipped it in alcohol to clean it, and then I . . . I stuck it in."

We helped her up onto the table and I started to examine her. She was pretty well along in the process of aborting, and as I introduced my fingers, I inadvertently broke the bag of waters. Alcohol on coat hangers must have a selective antibacterial effect: it must kill the harmless germs and leave only the real doozies. I won't even try to describe the odor that spread outward from that examining cubicle, but suffice it to say that, within three minutes, the chief resident was in the room to see what in the name of God had happened. He had been sitting in his office, a hundred yards away, around a corner, and with his door closed.

The woman did survive and went back to her Indiana home. There, she is most likely spending the rest of her days as the exemplary wicked maiden lady whose behavior should serve as a negative model for local damsels.

A woman worthy of mention was one who came to Bellevue for a relatively minor complaint, a nondescript vaginal itch. I was examining her when I noticed that the nurse was making wild gestures in the direction of the floor. She was pointing frantically in the direction of the patient's knitting bag, which was lying on the floor near the head of the examining table. From where the nurse was standing, she could see into the bag, but I couldn't. So, after I had finished the examination, I walked up to the head of the table and glanced sideways.

My God, it was right out of Edgar Allen Poe by way of Vincent Price. The bag was chock-full of the lady's instruments of trade. She had specula, uterine sounds, cervix grabbers, curettes, catheters, you name it. And dirty! The curettes were rusty and bloodstained. The catheters and specula had crud all over them. They looked as though they had never been washed. I thought the engraving on some of them looked familiar, so I bent over and picked out one of the specula, holding it as though it were carrying plague bacilli. Sure enough, it read, CITY OF NEW YORK, DEPT. OF HOSPITALS.

No wonder I hadn't been able to find a cause for this woman's problem as stated. She had been coming in with phony complaints to different GYN facilities, and when she had been left alone to dress or undress, she'd filled her knitting bag with various instruments she could use for abortions. There was a woman who who really stuck to her knitting.

She looked at me and I looked at her. I felt calm and prepared for any eventuality. Had she pulled a knife or a gun, I'd have promptly dropped the speculum back into the bag and offered her her choice of our stock of shiny new equipment. But she didn't say a word—just stared at me. Finally, I came out with, "What do you get for a job?"

She smiled sweetly. "Fifty bucks, Doc," she said. "And seventy-five or even a hundred if it's some snotty little college girl who's too afraid to tell her daddy."

"At those prices, don't you think you ought to at least wash your instruments?" I asked.

She stopped smiling and snapped at me, "Sheet, Doc, as long as you bastards won't do 'em nohow, you ain't got nuthin' to say. You hear me—NUTHIN'!" She glared harder. "Long as women want 'em and you won't do 'em, you're gonna keep me right in business." Then her expression relaxed, and she smiled again. "And I'll tell you, Doc," she added, "business is mighty, mighty good, too."

During the past few years, I've derived considerable pleasure from thinking of the severe business setback that woman has suffered since the Supreme Court ruling. But meanwhile, the Right to Life campaign to make time march backward continues. And I'm willing to bet more than a little money that I know one person who is eagerly watching that campaign, hoping it will soon bring the day when she'll once again be able to send the Bellevue gynecologists some of their most challenging cases. I'd also wager that the knitting bag is in her closet, full to overflowing with hardware and ready to go to work at a moment's notice. I'd even bet she still hasn't washed those damned instruments.

13

Come Quick, Doc,
He's Dead

During the early 1960's, one of the favorite pastimes of the Bellevue house staff was to get together every week and watch Ben Casey, that old TV show about a neurosurgical resident with all the human virtues of a tortured mongoose. We'd crowd around the set and hoot at the stupidity that the credulous public cheerfully swallowed as reality. The scenes that set off the largest numbers of outraged howls were the ones in which Ben, or one of his colleagues, rode in an ambulance to the scene of a disaster, and then heroically kept the patient alive as the vehicle screamed its way back to the hospital—not a moment too soon.

Thus, most people think they know about riding the ambulance: how the intern flies out of the Emergency Room and leaps onto the side of the vehicle. Then, holding the outside rail, his white coat flapping in the breeze, he risks life and limb as they zip through the city traffic. All this is presumably done so that when they reach the victim, the doctor may save one or two seconds getting to him. Such an intern would have to be more than a trifle tetched.

In actual fact, hospital-based ambulance calls have now pretty much gone by the boards. Certainly, interns don't go on the runs any longer: it's a dreadful waste of manpower. Besides, there are currently private and civil ambulance services which maintain vehicles stocked with first-class resuscitation equipment and staffed with paramedical attendants whose knowledge of first-aid procedures make the average intern look like a refugee from kindergarten. But back in my own internship days, we still took a turn going out to answer the calls. It was, though, very different from what was seen on Ben Casey.

The truth was, most of our ambulance runs were pretty tame affairs. For one thing, the genuine emergencies were already being attended to by prototype paramedicmobiles. Mostly we went out to get people who simply had no other means of transportation. Some were poverty-stricken elderly citizens who didn't have fifteen cents to spend on a bus. Others had the fifteen cents, but figured why the hell should they wait fifteen minutes in the rain on a street corner. Other calls were for people who had stopped breathing, whose hearts had stopped beating, and who were no longer moving. Of course, there was nothing anyone could do for them, but the gawkers standing around gnawing off their fingernails needed a specially trained individual in a white coat to tell them that the guy was officially dead. Then they could relax and go home to eat dinner.

Actually, we enjoyed going out on ambulance calls. Since we worked thirty-six hour stretches in the hospital, this was our one chance to get out for a while. Can you imagine that: a bunch of people who opted for breathing the New York City air because they considered it an improvement? That tells you something about what lack of sleep will do for a person's judgment. Or how thoroughly depressing Bellevue was. Or both.

An ambulance call usually began when someone happened to notify the police. They, in turn, would radio in to the ambulance dispatcher at The Vue. It was this worthy's job to get a crew together: a driver, an attendant, and the next intern "up." The three of us would climb into the meat wagon, strap ourselves securely in, and off we'd go to God-knows-what. Usually the essence of the requesting call bore little resemblance to what we'd actually find. But we often did get to meet some very interesting people on these runs.

One day we got a call to a fancy office building on Park Avenue South. As we wheeled up, the cop from the car parked in front of the building waved us to pull in next to him. As we leaped out of the back of the meat wagon, he yelled, "Thirty-second floor, Doc, hurry up." We ran on into the lobby.

When we got to the thirty-second floor, we encountered hordes of popeyed people, all pointing at and urging us toward one particular suite, whose door was open and from which issued the most piercing wails. We looked at one another. The attendant said, "Lawd, sounds lahka buncha god-damn ban-shees." The stretcher-bearer and I shrugged, and we all walked in.

The anteroom we entered was occupied by five or six women who were running about, apparently in random fashion, and periodically emitting the wails that we had heard from the hallway. One of them noticed us and motioned us frantically into the inner office. There we found a gentleman in his mid-forties. He was wearing a gray suit and was sprawled between a desk and a chair. His skin was bluish-gray and his pants were wet. It was obvious that he had been transferred to the Great Corporation in the Sky. I walked back into the anteroom, where I triggered off another burst of wailing. I asked if anyone could tell me what had happened.

The calmest member of the group, a tall, middle-aged woman who had been sitting at the desk dabbing at her eyes, came up to me. "I was taking dictation from him," she said, "when he just stopped talking and grabbed his chest, and turned gray all over, and slid out of his chair."

"How long ago did it happen?" I asked.

"About three o'clock," she answered. I looked at my watch; it was 3:40. At that point, a fat, heavily made-up woman ran over from the periphery where she had been pacing, and grabbed on to my lapels. "He's dead, isn't he?" she wailed.

"Well, uh . . . yes . . ."

That set her siren going full blast. "You don't have to tell me; I just know he's dead." She began to cry unconsolably.

I tried to calm her down. Aside from the commotion she was causing, she was on the verge of ripping my coat or choking me. "Was he your boss?" I asked her.

She looked up. "Oh no, I work in the office three doors down." She began to wail again.

"Well, was he a . . . er . . . a . . . friend of yours?"

"No, no, no, I never met him in my life. But he's dead, he's dead. Why the hell are you asking me all these questions, anyway?"

I unpried her from my collar and wondered why the hell I *was* asking her all those questions, anyway. I had heard of people who made a hobby of going to funerals, but I had always assumed that they were little old ladies with tennis sneakers, long black coats, and scraggly gray hair. I still wonder about this particular woman and her display of grief. Did she lead such a lonely, drab life that the opportunity to exhibit an emotion—any emotion at all—was irresistible? Maybe she just took John Donne a bit too seriously. In any event, we dispensed tranquilizers all around and told the women it might be well for them to go home. The hysterical interloper went back to her own office, and the other four women (all of whom had worked for the deceased) ran and hid in the ladies' room while we carried out the corpse. I've never been able to quite figure out why people do that, but they always do. I've asked psychiatrists about it, but since they all give me different answers, I don't think they really know either.

Another time that I was called out to care for a dead man, I ended up at a ritzy midtown restaurant. Here there was much less commotion. It was lunch hour, and the place was packed. The owner met us at the door and quickly and quietly ushered us in. It really was a first-class joint. The music was coming through the speakers at just the right volume so as not to disturb the muffled, genteel conversation.

Right from the beginning, the owner aroused my hostility. He was a thin little guy with a bald head and a monk's fringe. He wore a tuxedo and a pair of shoes that had a mirror-like shine. As he led me through by the least conspicuous path, he chattered incessantly at me in a stage whisper which he periodically interrupted in order to kowtow to one customer or another. It went like this:

"Oh, Doctor, I am so glad you are here. Yes, so very, very glad. Terrible—Yiz, Mrs. Jackson, so glad to see you again, my dear— terrible, terrible thing, the poor— Why, Mrs. Stanley, I see you've ordered the boeuf bourguignon. A very wise choice. Enjoy it, my dear—poor fellow, just keeled right over, and there was nothing— Good afternoon, Mrs. Danbury. Your presence honors my establishment—nothing at all to do, nothing at all. Could faint— Bon appetit, Mrs. Allison, heh heh heh—could just faint, Doctor."

Could just vomit, Owner, I thought. Fortunately, at this point, we had reached our destination. My little guide had led me to a table in a rear corner of the restaurant. It was sheltered by a screen; he pushed me behind it, and then followed me.

Three men were at the table. They were elderly, and very distinguished looking, all wearing dark suits with vests. Two of them were alive. The third was slumped in his chair, and he was very dead. Even in that condition, his face had a kindly look on it. Suddenly, I got an uncomfortable feeling, one of uncertain recognition. I pulled the man's wallet out of his pocket and looked inside. I had indeed recognized him. He was one of the older clinical professors at the medical school, at the time semiretired, and held in the highest regard by the faculty and students.

All the while, the owner had been standing behind me, wringing his hands and whispering how terrible, terrible this all was, really. When I straightened up, he took hold of my sleeve and stood up tall on his hind legs, so he could whisper conspiratorially into my ear. "I say, Doctor, I do hope you will be able to take him out the back door." He pointed out past the kitchen, into a narrow little alleyway, filled with garbage barrels and lined with broken glass and empty wine bottles. "We just can't have him going through the restaurant, can we? I'm sure you understand." He punctuated his request with his extra-special, deeply concerned expression.

"Sorry," I said sharply. "The stretcher won't fit out that way."

"But, Doctor, perhaps your attendant could just drag him . . ."

"Shut up," I answered, "and get out of the way."

I suppose I really should have gone out the back door—some of the diners did turn a little pale as we went along. But the good doctor did not leave the restaurant with the garbage, and I thought that was as it should have been.

A call I remember very well took me to one of those apartment houses between First Avenue and the East River, in the seventies. For the information of those who may live west of the Hudson River, that happens to be very expensive territory. The doorman let us in, told us the apartment number, and indicated the elevator to us. His tone and manner let us know what he thought of allowing Bellevue personnel into *his* building. Shithead, I thought, I know where you go when your belly hurts—and it ain't Harkness Pavilion.

We went up the elevator and down the hall, and then I had my one and only firsthand exposure to the way the really rich live in New York.

We walked through the door, and as we hit the carpet, I jumped. You've heard of the kind of rug you sink into up to your knees? Well, when I looked down, I literally could not see my shoes. Besides the entrance foyer, the place had a living room, a formal dining room, a bathroom, and a bedroom. You walked from the entryway down into the living room or up into the bathroom. I still can't fathom the significance of that. The floor in every room except the bathroom was covered with the same thick, green carpet, and the bathroom had ceramic tile. All the rooms, including the bathroom, were covered with that three-dimensional wallpaper that is supposed to be more expensive per unit weight than platinum. Crystal chandeliers were all over the place. The furniture looked like the stuff in museums that has cards on it and ropes across it to keep people from sitting down. And the bathroom fixtures: the sinks were genuine marble, and I thought the faucet handles were brass. That is, until I saw the little 14K marker engraved on each one.

The owner of this assortment of trinkets and baubles was sprawled across her bed which, by the way, was a super-kingsize affair with an ornate brass headpiece, all mounted on a semicircular elevation in the middle of the bedroom. She was as cold as a flounder. She had on an expensive nightgown that made me think of Chantilly and *peau de soie* and words like that. It contrasted weirdly with her false teeth, which were dangling halfway out of her mouth. She must have been in her seventies, Sir Somebody-or-other's widow. A picture of a young man in a recent-vintage army suit stood on her night table, and right next to the photo was a bottle of nitroglycerin tablets, prescribed by one of the Park Avenue specialists. This time, the pills hadn't worked.

While I was checking her over, the attendant was slowly going from room to room, taking it all in with a gaping jaw. Like me, he had never before seen a place like this. Finally, he came into the bedroom and let out a low whistle of awe alloyed with respect. "God damn, Doc!" he stage-whispered. "These people sure as hell die in style, don't they?"

The omega to the aforegoing alpha was my call to a run-down building in the mid-forties where we were met by the palest pair of policemen I've ever seen. "The guy on the third floor, looks dead in bed," one gasped. "Sure don't envy you."

"Whatsa matter?" I asked.

"Oh, Doc," said the other cop, wide-eyed. "I ain't never smelled nuthin' like that in my life."

I smiled condescendingly. Smells had never made me ill, and I assured them I'd be okay. They shook their heads and I galloped up to the third floor.

When I entered the room, I couldn't believe my senses. I gagged, and then retched. Quickly, I clamped my handkerchief over my nose. The best way I can describe the odor would be to ask you to imagine an airtight room in which a thousand dead armadilloes had been left for a year with large numbers of appropriate putrefactive bacteria. There were piles of junk all over the place, and in the far corner was what looked like an eighty-pound Rip Van Winkle lying in a bedspring. I said in, not on, because he was totally entangled in it. As I looked at him, he went, "Oooooeeeeeeeeeaaaaahhhhh," and feebly waved one hand in the air.

I beat it out the door and stood in the hallway, bracing myself against the wall. When I recovered sufficiently to go back downstairs, the cops were very nice. Neither one made a wisecrack, and they both asked me if I was all right. I said I was, and then choked out, "He's alive."

The cops turned pale all over again, and one asked whether I were certain. I said I had heard the old man groan and had seen him move.

"Well," opined the older cop, "you sure as hell can't work on him there."

I allowed that I was in total agreement.

Without another word, the officers went down to their car and returned a minute later, each wearing a gas mask. They picked up the old man, bedspring and all, and carted him down the three flights of stairs to the sidewalk. There, we tried to get him out of the bedspring, but we couldn't. To this day, I have no idea how that poor old man had managed to get himself so entangled in that bedspring. Finally, the cops got a couple of pairs of wire cutters and snipped the prisoner out. We loaded him into the meat wagon, and off we went to The Vue.

The old man died the next day. He had widespread tuberculosis and God knows what else. I called the super in his building to see whether he had a next of kin.

"I dunno," said the super. "Lived here 'bout twenny years, an' never saw nobody with 'im. Fact, ain't seen 'im at all for the las' two months. After y' left today, I went up an' searched 'is room—y' know, I figgered maybe he was one a them ol' guys with a million or so stashed away—"

"How did you stand the smell?" I asked.

"Din't notice no smell," he answered. "Anyways, din't find nuthin' but ol' magazines 'n' lotsa junk. So I t'rew it all out." He paused a moment, and then added brightly, "Say, Doc, y' know someone wants an apartment I'd appreciate y' sent 'im over."

Before I could answer, he added, "An' oh yeah—if y' do find a relative , wouldja tell 'im the sonovabitch owed me t'ree months rent?"

All the time I was going on ambulance calls, I kept waiting for an obstetrical emergency. By that time of the internship year, I had decided to go into obstetrics, and I was just itching to deliver a baby in an ambulance. During my last week on ambulance runs, the call came. We sped down to the Lower East Side, where a young girl had telephoned that her mother was having strong labor pains.

We arrived to find a Puerto Rican woman who weighed at least three hundred pounds writhing and rolling around on a bed in a one-room apartment. There were six kids clustered around her, and the oldest, who identified herself as Teresa, informed me that there were four more outside somewhere. She also said that her mother's pains had begun two hours before, and that they had become progressively worse. I sent the kids out into the hallway and examined the woman vaginally; it was apparent that she was not about to deliver. Somewhat disappointed, I told her we'd go to the hospital.

"No, no. No hospeetahl," she said.

I quickly painted pictures of hemorrhage, infection, seizures, death, and other terrors of unattended deliveries. Between mental and physical coercion, the two attendants and I got her up and ready to go. We called the public health nurse to look after Teresa and the other nine kids, and off we went. We got as far as the hallway when our patient squatted, pushed, and dropped a load of liquid stool on the floor. "Ay, bendito," she moaned, as she clutched her belly.

Christ, I thought, she must be about to deliver. So I checked her again. Still no sign that the baby was coming.

As we were getting into the ambulance, she clutched her abdomen, doubled over, cried, "Ay Dios mio," and decorated the street. We hastily pushed her into the ambulance, and I repeated the examination. Still no baby.

I was beginning to get concerned. I felt her abdomen to see if the uterus was showing signs of labor abnormalities, but she was so fat I couldn't feel the uterus at all. Shortly before we arrived at The Vue, she dropped Act Three in the ambulance. Another pelvic exam was as unrevealing as the others.

We rushed her onto a stretcher and zoomed up to the labor room. I hurriedly repeated my story to the obstetrical resident, and he examined the patient. Then, slowly turning to face me, he said wearily. "She's just got the shits. Her uterus is normal size; she's not even pregnant.

I began to splutter. "But . . . but . . . her daughter said—"

The resident put his hand on my shoulder. "Listen, you stupid bastard," he said quietly. "When it comes to pregnant women, I'd have hoped you'd know a little more than a fourteen-year-old kid."

14

All the Monkeys Weren't in the Zoo

Where to live was a major problem for most of the Bellevue house officers. The neighborhood around The Vue was in flux, and the choice of accommodations lay pretty much between a new apartment, which was well beyond the means of the average intern, and a rattrap in a building at least as old as Bellevue, which one of the justly renowned New York landlords might permit a young doctor to rent for $150 a month.

Some Bellevuers solved the dilemma by floating loans to be paid back when they entered practice. Others commuted an hour or more from New Jersey or Long Island. To a large number of the house staff, though, the answer was Stuyvesant Town.

Stuyvesant Town was (and still is) an apartment complex bounded by First Avenue, Avenue C, Fourteenth Street, and Twenty-third Street. It was built and maintained by the Metropolitan Life Insurance Company. The apartment units were large, clean, and light. The grounds were well kept, and had real grass and trees. In addition to this, the rentals were ridiculously low, ranging from about $80 to $125 a month.

Considering these facts, Stuyvesant Town was a popular place. New Yorkers by the droves sent applications for apartments, and then literally spent years on a waiting list. When and if they made it, they stayed. I met a man who lived there with his wife and teen-aged daughter; he told me that he figured he finally had it made, since his wife and he would be able to spend the remainder of their days in Stuyvesant Town. The thought made me feel nauseated, but this guy was beaming as befitted one who had been given the keys to his kingdom.

For some reason, the Lords of Stuyvesant Town looked with

favor on the Bellevue house staff. My wife and I sent in an application while we were paying $115 a month for the privilege of sharing three rooms with a brigade of cockroaches on East Nineteenth Street. Just nine months later, we moved to Stuyvesant Town, leaving the frozen water pipes and the vermin behind for the next lucky pair of newlyweds. Unbelievably, our new rent was only $88 a month.

Naturally there had to be a catch. Before we moved in, we were carefully screened. Then we signed a statement promising to abide by a long and complex set of rules and regulations, all aimed at maintaining the loveliness of the buildings and grounds. The list of thou shalt nots was impressive: walk on grass, slam doors, paint walls, install appliances and appurtenances (whatever they were), keep animals on the premises, and on and on literally for pages. My friend Mike Zimmerman, who also lived in Stuyvesant Town, summed it up one day by telling me that in his building, the residents were allowed to engage in sexual intercourse only on alternate Tuesdays and Thursdays.

Stuyvesant Town apartments were arranged in a linear fashion: our kitchen, dining area, living room, bathroom, and bedroom all opened off the right of a hallway that ran the length of the apartment. Only the coat closet opened to the left, right opposite the bathroom. Next door to each apartment was a mirror-image unit.

The inhabitant of our mirror-image was named Lizzie. At least, that's what Myra, my wife, and I called her. The name on her door plate read Elizabeth Oursley.

Lizzie was about fifty-five, tall, and gray-haired. Any way you looked at her, she was all angles, skinny and sticking out in every direction. She always wore a cotton-print dress. Her apartment was spotlessly clean and liberally adorned with antimacassars and glass and plaster figurines.

We first got to know Lizzie by post. One night while we were eating dinner, an envelope slid under the door and came to rest near Myra's feet. She tore it open and read it, and then began to laugh uproariously. "This is one of the funniest things I've ever seen," she spluttered, as the tears began to run down her cheeks.

"What is it?" I asked.

She brushed the tears away, and pushed the note across the table to me. It said:

APT 14:
In all fairness to yourselves and to myself I must ask
you to move your bed to the window end of your room.
I am sure I do not have to explain. Let me remind you
that these walls are paper thin and everything can be
heard.

APT 15

"What the hell is so funny?" I asked.

"It's a riot," choked my wife.

"Some riot. Of all the kooks in New York, I have to pick one to live next to who listens at the wall with a stethoscope."

"I hope she gets a charge."

"Well, I'm certainly not going to move my bed across the room and sleep under the window for her. Let *her* sleep under *her* window."

"Relax, dear," said Myra. "We'll probably never hear another thing about it."

It took me a while to get to sleep that night. Every time one of us turned over and a bedspring squeaked, my neck muscles tightened and I gnashed my teeth. By the time morning came around, I had conceived a thorough and heartfelt hatred for my keen-eared neighbor.

The next night I was on call at the hospital. Myra stayed with me to help with the laboratory work. We were busy, so rather than go home at 2 A.M., she slept the rest of the night in my hospital room. I was up all night, and by the following evening I was pretty irritable. After supper I was dozing in the living room when the phone rang. Myra was in the bathroom, so I answered it. A high, nervous voice with a slight quaver asked, "Is this Apartment 14?"

I allowed that it was.

"Well, this is Apartment 15."

I began to wake up.

"Did you get my note two nights ago?" asked the voice.

I said we had.

"Well, sir, I really do wish you would pay attention to it. Last night, your . . . your . . . your *cavortings* kept me up most of the night. I really don't want to make trouble, but I will not—"

"Just wait a minute, please," I interrupted. "Do you mean last night or the night before?"

"I mean *last night*. I know what I mean. And you know what I mean, too. And furthermore, I want to tell you that I will not tolerate this indecency! Do you understand?"

The question was rhetorical, because before I could get more than "urk" out, she had hung up with a slam. As I replaced the receiver, Myra walked in and asked who it was.

"It was Mrs. Apartment 15," I said. "She wanted to complain about our scandalous behavior last night."

"But we weren't home."

"I know. But she seems to think we were."

Myra looked puzzled. "Now what?" she asked.

"Christ, I don't know. Is she violent? Might she kill?"

Myra giggled. "Loony Lizzie took an ax and gave her neighbor forty whacks."

"Well," I said. "Maybe we ought to meet the lady. At least see what we're up against."

"You or me?"

"Both. Then, if she starts screaming or something, we'll be around to help each other."

"Should we call and invite her over some night?"

"You kidding? Let her in here? Let's go to her place. Now."

"Just walk over?"

"Sure, why not?"

Myra shrugged, and we went out the door and walked the six paces to Apartment 15. We knocked, and an eye appeared at the peephole. "Yes? What is it?" piped the phone voice.

"My name is Apartment 14, but my friends call me Laurence Karp," I said. "My wife and I want to talk to you." In retrospect, I think it's possible that I might have been showing a little hostility.

Lizzie opened the door and let us into her neat and ordered little world. I wondered whether there was a plaque hidden behind a sofa in memory of the last living bacterium in the apartment who had died a horrible death before the relentless epidemic of Mr. Clean.

I was not prepared for the reception we got. My stars, she was just terribly sorry to raise all that fuss, and really, we did look like such a lovely young couple, and she certainly did hope we understood how embarrassing it all was for her. Finally, she assured me that henceforth she would call me Mr. Karp, not 14, and that I was to feel free to address her as Mrs. Oursley. "Now," she beamed, "wouldn't you like a nice cup of tea?"

My wife and I had a sudden attack of Hanselandgretelitis, but despite a frantic exchange of stares and mouthings, we could think of no tactful way out. Mrs. Oursley put on the water and sat down.

I hemmed once and hawed a couple of times, and then, with all good tact and consideration, I introduced the major topic by informing our hostess that neither my wife nor I had been at home the previous evening.

"Well," she said, "I really don't understand that. I did hear something, you know."

Then she smiled at us. Sweetly. She looked just like anyone's dear little gray-haired mother. I know she didn't believe me. We had really been at home, had fornicated wildly and loudly and via every forbidden orifice, and now we were trying to pull the wool over her eyes.

At that point, she changed the subject. She chattered on for a half an hour or so about life as a lonely middle-aged woman in lovely Stuyvesant Town. I wondered whether or not there had ever really been a Mr. Lizzie. If so, he had long since passed to what had to be his just reward.

Later in the evening, as we left, Lizzie reminded us what lovely young people we were, and how she was just certain that there would be no more unpleasant misunderstandings. Those were the words she used.

About a week later, I came home from work, and found a letter addressed to Mr. Karp, Apt. 14. I ripped open the envelope and found a surprise. Rather than another circumlocutory assortment of euphemisms related to my satyrical pursuits, it was a plainly worded memorandum from one of the assistant managers of Stuyvesant Town, requesting that I meet with him two afternoons hence, in order that we might clarify some unpleasant misunderstandings.

My immediate impulse was to bash in the door at Apartment 15, beat the occupant to death with a figurine, and leave her wrapped in antimacassars on the assistant manager's office doorstep. However, I restrained myself. The cool-headed approach, I decided, would be better.

The next afternoon my wife told me she had gotten a phone call from the assistant manager. "But he wouldn't talk to me," she said. "He wanted to know if you had received his note."

"What did you say?"

"Oh, I played dumb. I asked him what he wanted, and what it was all about, and you should have heard him splutter. Finally, he just asked me to tell you he wants to see you at four o'clock tomorrow, and if you have any questions, you should feel free to call him."

"You really embarrassed the poor man."

"No, dear. He embarrassed himself. I didn't do a thing."

At four o'clock the next day, I went to the office of the assistant manager. He was the very model of an assistant manager in the early 1960's: about forty, balding, sweaty, with rimless glasses, and a habit of looking at his watch at approximately thirty-second intervals. I had the feeling that if I had asked him at mid-interval for the time, he'd have had to glance again before he'd have been able to tell me.

With a "Dr. Karp, I'm glad you could come," he showed me to a seat, and then proceeded to apologize profusely for having addressed my envelope to Mr. Karp. "That was the name I was given. I didn't realize you were a doctor until I, uh, checked your, uh, records here."

I assured him that I was neither crushed nor angered by his oversight, and that I could indeed find it in my heart to forgive him.

"Uh, let me come to the point, uh, Dr. Karp. It's about your neighbor in 15—"

"Mrs. Oursley."

"Yes, of course, Mrs. Oursley. Uh, Dr. Karp, uh, the problem is, uh, Mrs. Oursley . . . uh, says, uh . . . ."

He paused and mopped his brow; he looked as though he were going to wring out his handkerchief in the wastebasket. I decided that the only decent thing to do was to put him out of his misery.

"Mrs. Oursley has been complaining that our nocturnal behavior is disturbing her," I said.

The assistant manager allowed himself a tentative smile. "Yes, Dr. Karp. That's well put." He glanced at his watch. "She says she has mentioned it to both you and your wife on several occasions, and has asked you to move your bed to the other end of the room. Now, that doesn't sound unreasonable, does it?"

"Actually, it does," I said. "For several reasons. First, it's too cold to sleep under the window. Furthermore, if we put the bed on any other wall, we'd have to walk across it to get to the other side of the room."

"But—"

"What's more, this lady hears noises when there are none."

"What do you mean?" He wiped his forehead, and then snuck a glance wristward.

"Because last Tuesday night she called to tell me that we had kept her up the whole night before. I was at the hospital for the whole night. What's more, just to keep the issues straight, my wife spent the entire night with me at the hospital. And furthermore, I can assure you, we did not give another couple the key to our place. In short, our apartment was empty that night."

The assistant manager looked stricken. I could see the little men with hammers begin to whack at his temples. "Oh, I was afraid it was something like that again," he whimpered.

"Like what—again?" I whimpered back.

"Oh, Dr. Karp, it's just terrible. Last year, we had something very much like this happen. A man—a very nice man—lived in the building next to yours, and the woman who lived in the apartment downstairs from him kept complaining to us that he was making obscene advances to her. He denied ever having spoken to her. In fact, he said he had never even noticed her. She called us every day; one time it would be a proposition in the hall, and the next, an obscene phone call. We just didn't know what to do."

Yes indeedy, I thought. In Stuyvesant Town, you really can't tell the players without a scorecard. But I smiled sympathetically, and he went on.

"Well, I'll tell you, we were really in a spot. Finally, one day, she rang his doorbell without a stitch of clothing on."

I guffawed. I couldn't help it. "Stark raving nude?" I asked.

He looked a bit sternly at me, and then checked the hour, minute, and second. "Uh . . . yes, yes. She began to claw at him, and was screaming 'Rape me, rape me, goddamnit.' Or something like that. Fortunately, one of the other neighbors saw the whole thing and called the police, and they took her off."

At that point I had it made, and I knew it. I scratched my head and mused, "Well, that is frightening. Actually, I *have* been a bit worried about my wife's safety when I've been away. As you know, I work at night a lot."

"Oh yes, I can imagine an intern's lot is not pleasant."

He really had checked me out thoroughly. "Yes, we work every other night. And while I'm down here talking to you, the fellow who was on call all last night is doing my work and his too. Then, when I do get home, I have to put up with these notes and phone calls." I was almost shouting; I had myself convinced how angry I was. "I do hope this will be the end of the matter."

"I'm sure it will be, Dr. Karp." 4:17:41. "I will speak to Mrs. Oursley and tell her that I'm convinced that there is nothing more that you can do to accommodate her, and that she must not disturb you further, or we will have to ask *her* to vacate."

I said my thanks and left him drying off his forehead, undoubtedly trying to remember what insane impulse had led him to major in business administration and not in something reasonable like veterinary medicine.

About a week and a half later I was spending the night at The Vue when, about midnight, a patient was admitted to my service. She was a feeble, eighty-seven pound, eighty-seven-year old, white-haired lady who was totally out of it. To any question I put to her, she only smiled sweetly and patted me on the hand and arm. She had been sent in from her nursing home with an admission diagnosis of fecal impaction, which seemed like a hell of a reason for a midnight admission, but at Bellevue the unusual was commonplace. Seeing the futility of trying to take a history, I patted her back on the arm and began to do a physical examination. I didn't get far. Her pulse was thready, rapid, and terribly irregular. So I quickly checked her heart and lungs, which made it clear that she was going into heart failure. Hooking her up to an electrocardiograph machine, the cause showed itself to be a severe heart attack. All the usual therapeutic procedures for heart attacks and failure didn't seem to do anything for her, but she appeared to be comfortable. Then, I began to wonder whether her apparent senility was really only the result of a temporary oxygen deficiency in the brain as a result of the heart attack—that sometimes does happen. So I looked up the phone number of the nursing home, called the place, and got connected with the nurse on my patient's former floor. I identified myself and asked her whether she remembered Mrs. O'Leary.

"Sure do," she answered. "We bofe bin here a loooooong time, her and me t'gether. Ah wuz s'prised not t' see her tonight."

"What I need to know," I went on, "is what her mind was like. Was she sort of out of things—senile—when she was with you?"

The nurse laughed raucously. "Lawd," she said. "That pore li'l ol' lady ain't said a word y' could make sense outa in years. But she shore is sweet."

I agreed that she did seem very nice.

"Whutsamatta wif Miz O'Leary, anyway?"

"Looks like kind of a bad heart attack."

She knew. After years as graveyard-shift nurse in a nursing

home, you learn. She didn't ask me whether or not Mrs. O'Leary would be okay. She just said, "Keep 'er cumftable, now, heah?"

I said I would, and thanked her very much. I went back to the bed where Mrs. O'Leary was dozing. I'd do what I could, but now if it didn't work, I wouldn't have to feel so bad.

She remained stable through the night, not short of breath, constantly smiling and patting. About 6 A.M. she suddenly worsened; you could see the cardiograph tracings of the heartbeats slowly but progressively became smaller and farther apart. She still was smiling and breathing easily, but she was getting drowsier and her irrelevant words gave way to unintelligible mutterings. Her blood pressure was falling. Nothing that the cardiology consultant or I tried did any good. A little after 7 o'clock she blew a couple of bubbles from her lips and turned blue. The cardiograph line stayed level. It happened so gradually, it really seemed hard to do anything as definite and well-defined as to pronounce her dead, but that was part of the job, so I did it.

Her original admission slip had listed no next of kin, but our experience with New York City nursing homes being what it was, I waited till 8 A.M. and then called the office of the home's director. I explained that I was pretty sure that his establishment had not been housing and feeding Mrs. O'Leary unless some next of kin had been footing the bill. He snappishly said he'd check his records and put me onto the hold line. Some people just have no sense of humor.

A minute later, he cut back in. "Doctor," he barked. "The next of kin is her daughter, Mrs. Elizabeth Oursley, who lives at . . . "

He read off the address and phone number, but I didn't listen, since I knew them very well. I thanked him and hung up.

A minute or two later, my co-intern, Gerald Sanders, walked in. "Another all-nighter?" he grinned. "Christ, you look awful."

I grabbed him by the tie. I actually did. "You've got to help me, Gerry," I croaked. I rapidly told him the story of Loony Lizzie and her erotic nocturnal delusions. "My God, Gerry, I can't call her now," I said. "She'd really go off the deep end."

"You want me to call her?"

"Yes, and sign the death certificate."

Notifying the relatives was probably the least favorite job of an intern. None of us had yet accumulated enough experience with grief-stricken, guilt-ridden relatives to be anything but acutely uncomfortable in this circumstance.

Gerry grimaced. "What's it worth to you?" he asked.

"I'll tell you what it's worth—to you. You won't have it on your conscience that you're responsible for sending some poor nutty lady to the hatch. And furthermore, if she decides to kill me, you'll have to work every single night for the next month."

"Come on, Larry, she's not that bad."

"Haven't you worked at Bellevue long enough yet, Gerry?" I stared at him.

"Jesus Christ," he muttered. "All right. I'll call her."

Gerry called her, and she came right over to the hospital. I hid in the sleeping quarters until he returned to tell me that she had left. I asked him how she had taken it.

"Fine, Larry. She just said she'd been kind of expecting it for a while, and her mother was so senile anyway. She thanked me and left. No tears or anything."

"God, I wouldn't have believed it."

"She seemed perfectly okay to me, Larry." He grinned again. "The way I figure it, maybe you really ought to move your bed."

A couple of months went by, and all was quiet from the direction of Apartment 15. I thought that it was over, once and for all. Then, one night, after another all-night stand at The Vue, I was slumped on the bed, absorbing the night's supply of pap from the tube. Folks were singing and dancing and telling jokes, and I was almost asleep. Then the phone rang, and my wife picked it up. She called out, "It's for you." I reached over and said hello.

"Mr. Karp, this is Mrs. Oursley. I have something I'd like to ask you about."

Omigod, I thought, she found out. She thinks I killed her mother. "Yes . . . yes?"

"Mr. Karp, I just wonder: do you have a motor running in your bedroom."

I briefly considered asking her whether her real worry was that I had managed to invent automated coitus, but I decided not to. I merely assured her that there was no motor in our bedroom, that we were peacefully watching television, and that there was only singing, dancing, and joke-telling coming over the airways. No motors. I even offered to permit her to inspect the premises.

"Oh no, Mr. Karp, that won't be necessary. I just wanted to check. It sounds like . . . like there's an *airplane* in your bedroom. That's all."

"Well, there's no airplane in the bedroom, Mrs. Oursley. You know they don't allow them in Stuyvesant Town apartments."

"Oh, certainly, Mr. Karp. I just wanted to check. Thank you."
With that, she hung up.

That episode was, in fact, the end of it. For the remaining year
and a quarter that we lived in Stuyvesant Town, I neither saw nor
heard from Lizzie again. But ever since we moved out, I've often
felt the urge to call the present occupant of Apartment 14 to ask
him whether anyone has been taking auditory exception to his
unconscionable lasciviousness. However, I've never been able to
get myself to do it. Probably in 1964, there was a guy somewhere
who never quite had the nerve to call me and ask me the same
question.

15

Visitations at The Vue

Generally speaking, hospitals aren't exactly what you'd call wide-open institutions. In fact, their security systems probably are exceeded only by those of federal penitentiaries. Even at that, it's close.

For example, consider what's involved in paying a visit to your Aunt Martha while she's recovering from her hysterectomy at your community hospital. As you go through the revolving door into the glistening lobby, you barely get past the entry to the gifte shoppe when you hear a squeaky, "May I help you, sir?" You turn to see two little old ladies wearing cotton dresses and snappy volunteer caps, sitting behind a rectangular wooden table. One of them looks like your grandmother, and the expression on the face of the other suggests that you made her an indecent proposal.

You walk up to the table and explain your mission, whereupon your grandmother smiles benignly and begins to rummage through a shoebox in front of her. "I'm sorry," she finally says. "But her cards are all out."

Your heart jumps into your throat as you wonder whether Grandma meant to say that Aunt Martha has cashed in her chips. But then she goes on to explain that patients are allowed two visitors at a time, and that each is given a card to use as a sort of hall pass. "If you'll have a seat over there," she says, gesturing across the lobby, "I'll call you when one of her visitors comes down." Meanwhile, the other old bird is giving you a look calculated to straighten out any potential sinner who might even consider the possibility of exhausting a poor recuperating woman by becoming her third simultaneous visitor.

You sit down on an unpadded wooden chair and, within fifteen

151

minutes, you feel like a candidate for disk surgery. You try to take your mind off the pain that's shooting down the back of your legs by leafing through a year-old copy of *Time* magazine, but it doesn't help. Carefully, you stand up, and cautiously, you take a few steps. Hands behind your back, you try to get interested in the stuffed animals and boxes of candy in the windows of the gifte shoppe. You try to calculate the average number of colored splotches in each square of the tile floor.

After an endless three-quarters of an hour, Grandma summons you over, gives you your hall pass, and sends you toward the elevators. Before you can go up, the burly elevator operator checks to be sure you've been officially sanctioned. The surveillance is repeated by the nurse on Aunt Martha's floor, who then makes certain you go into the proper room. Just checking to see that there's no sneaking in of any unauthorized visiting to other patients.

Ten minutes after your arrival, Aunt Martha is in the middle of an animated speech extolling the manifold advantages of a spayed existence when the nurse comes in to tell you that visiting hours are over and you will have to leave. Cut off more sharply than she was from her generative organs, Aunt Martha voices her disappointment, whereupon the nurse tells her that patients must get their rest, and it's really too bad that her visitor (as she looks at you balefully out of the corners of her eyes) has been so inconsiderate as to come so late in the day. Then she personally escorts you from the room, making it clear that the thoughtlessness which set off the little sermon has cost your aunt a precious and irreplaceable forty-five seconds of repose.

At The Vue, however, that's not quite the way it worked. Although there were flyspecked signs posted on various walls to announce the proper visiting periods, no one paid much attention to them. At the end of visiting hours, a voice would announce that fact over the loudspeaker system, but the innumerable bedside chats went on as before. If there happened to be a nurse or an aide on the ward, she might try to personally reinforce the message, but her plea would almost inevitably turn out to be a cry in the wilderness. Visitors came and left at will, as well as in unregulated numbers. More than once on afternoon rounds, we had to claw our way to a patient's bedside through a solid pack of children, parents, brothers, sisters, aunts, uncles, nieces, nephews, spouses, lovers, and neighborhood kibitzers. Then we'd have to shoo them all away to a distance that would allow us to examine the patient and discuss his prognosis and therapy.

Nor did patients at The Vue get nearly as much rest as did their counterparts in private hospitals. Frequently, a family would bring dinner for a shut-in, and for themselves as well. Some nights, you could have closed your eyes and been in any rib emporium on the West Side. We often had to make late-night rounds to pick up the half-empty Malta Corona bottles and uneaten pieces of fried chicken, lest some patient be trampled to death by the stampede of rats and *cucarachas* which otherwise surely would have ensued.

The reason for the freedom of movement in The Vue was as much a function of the topography of the hospital as of understaffing. Physically as well as conceptually, Bellevue was an open building. No barriers, structural or human, existed to impede the flow of visitor traffic. To gain access to the wards, one didn't even have to go through the lobby. There were several wide, parallel corridors which led directly to stairs to the ward areas. Even in the lobby itself, though, there were no obstacles. The bums sleeping on the rows of benches couldn't have cared less who went where in the hospital.

So if you knew where your friend or relative was located, you simply walked through or around the lobby to the stairs or the elevators. If not, you went over to one of the information clerks, who were located on the left side of the lobby, behind a row of black-barred cages.

"Sadie Murphy's on Ward G-2," the clerk would growl at you. "Take them stairs over there up one flight and make a left. But you can't go up till visiting hours; that's two-thirty." Then the clerk would go back to her confession magazine, while you went up them stairs one flight and made a left.

Not all the visitors to The Vue were exactly what one might call friends and relatives. One day, my co-intern, Jack Thorn, called me over to say that he thought there was something peculiar about the grimy-looking small fellow who was visiting Mr. Rodriguez in the back of the ward. I looked the man over for a few minutes, and then shrugged my shoulders.

"I don't know," I said. "He doesn't look any more peculiar to me than anyone else here."

"There's something about him," Jack said, with a scowl. "I just can't put my finger on it."

During the next two days, Jack studied the little man. He would come in about midafternoon, walk directly to the back of the ward, and sit and talk with Mr. Rodriguez for perhaps fifteen minutes. Then he'd get up and walk out.

On the third day, Jack came up to me, all excited and agitated. "I've got it," he announced with finality. "I know who that bastard is."

I looked toward the back of the ward, where the visit was progressing according to schedule. "All right then," I said. "Who is he?"

Instead of answering my question, Jack asked me one. "What's Rodriguez here for?"

I think I must have looked at Jack a little sharply. "He's got hepatitis," I said. "And he's—"

Suddenly, at that point, the light began to dawn.

"—a junkie."

Jack smirked, and smugly nodded his head.

I glanced back at Mr. Rodriguez and his guest. "You think that guy's selling him drugs?" I asked. "You think he's a pusher?"

"I'm sure of it," Jack answered quickly. "I told you I thought there was something funny about him, and I just realized what it is. You remember Charlie Jackson, don't you?"

I made a face. It would be a long while before any of us on that ward would be able to forget Charlie Jackson. He was an addict who had been our patient a month before. With his filthy needles, he had injected bacteria into his blood stream. The bacteria then had proceeded to set up colonies on his heart valves, a condition known as acute bacterial endocarditis. It's not a very good thing to have even now, but in 1963 it was virtually 100 percent fatal. Charlie Jackson lingered for three weeks, gasping for breath in his oxygen tent. His last intelligible words were "Gimme methadone."

I assured Jack that I remembered Charlie Jackson very well indeed.

"Well, this same character used to visit Charlie every afternoon, too," said Jack. "That's where I know him from. And if I'm not wrong, he stopped visiting about the time Charlie became so weak it would have been impossible for him to give himself a fix."

"Son of a bitch!" I muttered. "No wonder Charlie's blood cultures stayed positive. He was shooting in the bugs as fast as we were running in penicillin."

"That's right," agreed Jack. We looked again toward the back of the ward, where at that moment the suspect was taking his leave of Mr. Rodriguez.

"I'm going to fix that little scumbag good," said Jack.

He did, too. The next morning, Jack went down and spoke to the captain of the guards, and at midafternoon, when the scrawny man walked onto the ward, two of the biggest guards took him by the arms and led him into the examining room. There, out of sight of all possible witnesses, they frisked him and found several bags of heroin which, we later found out, were just as dirty as they could be. That pusher was a walking disease vector, a Typhoid Mary of the first class. God only knows how many other addicts he made suffer and die like Charlie Jackson had. When the guards found the heroin on him, he began to squeak out his innocence, and then he protested that the guards had no right to strong-arm and search him. Perhaps because he knew that was true and it upset him, the larger of the two guards hauled off and clouted the pusher solidly in the solar plexus. Then he and his buddy dragged the white-faced, gasping man out and down to the local precinct house. I don't know whether he was eventually convicted, but I am quite certain he was never again seen plying his trade at The Vue.

Not only drugs were sold by Bellevue visitors. One evening I had to draw a blood sample from Mr. Harris, one of our long-term residents. He had been admitted for a particularly severe case of viral pneumonia, and for a while we all despaired of his leaving our ward any way other than feet first. But he proved to have considerable recuperative powers, and although it took a few weeks, he overcame his microbial invaders and was on the verge of discharge. As I approached Mr. Harris' bed with my needle and syringe, I noticed that the curtain was drawn, but I didn't think anything of the fact. Usually, this was nothing more than a sign that the patient wished to get a little sleep and the tumult on the ward was distracting him. So I strode up to the curtain and briskly threw it open. In the same motion, however, I even more briskly threw it shut, and more briskly yet walked away and into the examining room where I dropped my syringe and needle on the floor.

Mr. Harris hadn't been alone in his bed. There had been a young woman there with him, and what she was doing to Mr.

Harris—well, I used to try to tell people about it, but I've long since given up because it makes me stutter so badly no one can understand me. God Almighty, I didn't think the contortionists in the circus were capable of such feats.

Well, I decided I was going to just sit in the treatment room and pretend that the whole thing had never happened. Perhaps I might never come out. Certainly I wouldn't budge until the following afternoon, by which time Mr. Harris, and presumably his acrobatic guest, would be off the ward.

Not ten minutes later, though, as I was staring at the garbage scows on the East River, I was startled by a strident "Hey, Doc," from behind me in the doorway. I turned around to see Mr. Harris' lady friend standing there, wearing the most lecherous leer I've ever seen. If a face can possibly turn both red and white at the same time, I know mine did. I realized she required an acknowledgment, but I couldn't collect myself sufficiently to say, "Yes, what can I do for you?" Actually, maybe it's just as well I couldn't. In any event, I just stood there with my eyes and mouth wide open, staring at her.

She looked pretty much like your average New York hooker, in her early twenties, heavily made-up, with a goodly assortment of those black spots painted on her face, and none-too-neat jet-black hair hanging past her shoulders. Her skirt barely covered her gizzard.

Eventually she took my agitated silence for an answer of sorts, and waved her hand in what might have been a disparaging fashion. "Don't worry none about breakin' in on us like that, Doc," she said in her brassy street voice. "It ain't the first time I had guys watching me do my thing, and Bob, it didn't bother him, neither. Fact, he thought it was kinda funny."

I said something to the effect that I was glad to have been able to brighten Mr. Harris' day.

The leer disappeared from the woman's face. "Bob ain't gonna get in no trouble becuz of this, is he?" she asked.

"Oh, no," I said. "No. No, no, no, no." I had a brief, horrible vision of filling out an incident report on the matter. I was afraid that even my writing would stutter if I tried to do that.

"I wouldn't tell anyone here a thing about it," I said fervently.

The hooker smiled in relief. "Oh, that's good," she said. "Y'know, Doc, me and my friends work this place a lot. You got a buncha guys here, y'know, maybe they were sick bad when they came in, but then they get better, and, well, y'know, they get a little lonesome, and they can't wait till they get out. So my friends and me, we just cruise around the wards during the visiting hours, and when one of the boys gives us the signal, we go on over, pull the curtain, and go to work."

"How do you get paid?" I asked. "All their money's locked up in the hospital safe."

The leer returned. She pulled a little notebook out of her purse, and held it aloft for inspection. "We write down our jobs," she said. "Then, when the boys get out, we go and look them up. I won't say I never lost no money on a Bellevue trick, but no more'n I get shafted on the street."

"I guess it's warmer working the wards than the streets in wintertime, too," I said.

The leer changed into a genuine good-natured grin. "Yeah, that's for darn sure," the girl said. She turned to leave. "Be seeing you around, Doc. Thanks a lot," she called over her shoulder, as she went out the door.

Since that day, I've acquired a genuine respect for a closed curtain around a hospital bed. Respect, hell—it's close to being a phobia. I've never again opened a bed curtain, either on an open ward or in a private room, without first having announced my presence and requested permission.

Thus, some visitors to The Vue brought death with them, and others brought life. The strangest member of the former group was the woman I called the Crow.

I first noticed her one afternoon, a few days after I had been transferred onto B-2, one of the male medicine wards. She walked onto the ward at precisely two-thirty, the official starting time of visiting hours. She was tall, about five-nine, and very thin. Her most noticeable feature, though, was her clothing. She was wearing a floor-length black dress which swished around her ankles as she walked. Her mouth seemed to be frozen into just the smallest trace of a smile, which might have been described as a shit-eating grin. In combination with her dress and general appearance, however, it gave me the creeps. As she went past me, she set off a general wave of goose pimples on my body. I shook my head and figured I just hadn't been getting enough sleep.

She moved to a point approximately at the middle of the ward, and stood there a moment, looking around. Then her eyes fell on

Howard Runyon. Howard was a Bowery fellow who had partaken of the grape too hard and too long. First he had developed cirrhosis of the liver, and then liver cancer. Now, yellow and shrunken, he lay semicomatose in his deathbed.

The strange woman glided over to Howard and sat down noiselessly on a metal chair at the bedside. She took the dying man's hand in hers, and leaned over him, obviously whispering tender words of affection and comfort into his ear. For two hours, she continued to do so, and at four-thirty, when the loudspeaker announced the end of the visiting period, the woman kissed Howard lightly on his forehead, stood up, and walked silently off the ward, her facial expression unchanged.

This whole business surprised me. I hadn't known that Howard Runyon had had anyone in the world who cared about him, and certainly not anyone who looked like that. But life at The Vue was full of little surprises, and it seemed entirely reasonable that this was a girlfriend, or perhaps an estranged wife, temporarily come a bit unglued over Howard's obvious moribund condition. So I paid much less attention the next day when the entire act was repeated.

The night after the second visit, Howard Runyon died. After making the necessary official pronouncement, I went to check his next of kin. I did so with a good bit of uneasiness. The idea of having to call up that peculiar woman didn't appeal to me in the slightest. Hence I was both relieved and surprised to discover that Howard had no listed next of kin, and no one to call in case of emergency. I quickly got over the surprise: I knew very well that any Bowery relationships that do take place are noteworthy for their absence of formalities. But then I realized that I'd have to watch for Howard's visitor at two-thirty the next afternoon, and my relief passed along with my surprise.

The woman never showed up the next day, though, and it wasn't until the day after that that I saw her again. She had come onto the ward while I was busy, and it was about three when I noticed her at the bedside of Mr. Rosario, an octogenarian Puerto Rican whose kidneys had given up for good, and who was then in the terminal stages of uremia. Mr. Rosario was by no means a Bowery Bum: he was the head of a large and devoted family who came religiously to see him every evening. Yet here was this black-gowned female, holding his hand and crooning into his at-best semi-hearing ear.

Mr. Rosario looked nothing like Howard Runyon, but I

imagined that in her grief, perhaps the woman hadn't noticed the difference. She was unquestionably at least a little dippy, and we had, in fact, moved Mr. Rosario into Mr. Runyon's bed after the latter's departure.

As hard as I tried, I couldn't figure any way out of the situation, so I clenched my teeth and sidled over to the bedside. "Excuse me, Madam," I said, as I drew up. "I . . . I don't think you've noticed, but this isn't Mr. Runyon. It's Mr. Rosario. Mr. Runyon . . . er . . . well, died. Two nights ago."

She looked up at me with that same little smile on her face. "Oh, I know," she said. "Poor Mr. Runyon. It's so sad, isn't it? There's *so* much sadness in the world." She looked back at the bed, where Mr. Rosario's chest was slowly, rhythmically rising and falling. Her smile widened, ever so slightly. "And now, Mr. Rosario is going to die, too. Poor Mr. Rosario."

She turned back to Mr. Rosario, leaned over him, and whispered throatily, "But don't you worry, dear. It doesn't hurt at all. It's just like dropping off to sleep. Just as easy and natural as that." She patted his hand.

I quickly retreated to the front of the ward. The case of the creeps I had had upon first seeing that woman was a pleasant experience compared to what I felt now. I knew she was playing about as deep as possible in left field, but I still wasn't exactly sure what the game was.

That night, Mr. Rosario died, and two days later the Crow, as I had christened her, was giving solace to Mr. Clark as he was going down for the count from lung cancer. Three days after that, she moved on to Mr. Holley and his intractably failing heart. By then, I had all I could take. There was something obscene about the way the Crow would unerringly select the farthest-gone patient on the ward, visit with him for the brief time he had left, and then, after a decent day off to mourn for the dead, reappear to claim her next victim. I decided to go over to the psychiatry building and discuss the matter with my friend Sid Albright, who was a psych resident.

Sid listened to my speech, and then nodded and said, "Uh-huh."

"It makes sense to you?" I asked.

"I think so," said Sid. "Some people might say that this is a lady who happens to have it in for men, for some reason, and enjoys watching them die, but I think there's more to it than that. To me, it sounds like a type of necrophilia, a morbid fascination with corpses. It may even involve eroticism. Since dead bodies are a little hard for laymen to come by, sometimes these characters develop an attachment to the almost-dead." Sid looked thoughtful for a moment, and then continued. "I really think it's almost as though they suck their own vital energy from the dying; in a psychic sense they feed upon the moribund."

"So you think this lady must have figured a big city hospital would give her all the nourishment she could handle?" I asked.

Sid shrugged. "Who the hell knows how she got started coming here?" he said. "Maybe she really did come to visit a friend or a relative and saw how easy it would be to just keep coming. What difference does it make?"

"None, really," I answered. "Just tell me how to get rid of her, that's all."

Sid looked at me curiously. "Why do you want to do that?" he asked. I returned the curiosity with interest.

"Why?" I squeaked. "You think I should just leave this crazy necromaniac loose on the wards, to choose a new dying patient every day like you or I would pick out a cream puff?"

"I don't see why not," Sid said calmly. "When you come right down to it, what's she doing that's illegal? Or even immoral, for that matter? So she comes in and visits dying men. At least while she's there, they know that they're not alone and that someone cares about them while they're dying. That's more than they get from either you or me. So she gets a thrill from doing it. So what? If I were to analyze the reasons why you're in training to become a doctor it's entirely possible that no decent examining board would ever give you a license." He laughed.

"Very funny," I said. "I should have known better than to ask a Shrink for advice. I should have realized it'd be me who'd end up having perversions and a twisted mind."

"That's right," said Sid. "Feel good and guilty. Guilt is such a wonderful thing. If it weren't for guilt, psychiatrists all over the world would be starving."

I stomped back to the ward and kicked a large indentation into the metal wastebasket. At that moment, the Crow was savoring her current cream puff, a seventy-five-year-old man with a stroke and pneumonia. I felt an overwhelming urge to rush over, grab her by her neck, and pitch her out the nearest window into the parking lot two flights below. But then, I began to think about what Sid had said. That old stroke victim had been on the ward for two full weeks, and the Crow was the first and only visitor he had had. So I capitulated. Live and let live. Don't knock it till you've tried it. For the rest of my rotation on Ward B-2, I had twenty-four to forty-eight hours' notice when to throw in the towel on a patient. She proved to be an infallible prognosticator. But right up till my last day on the ward, she still gave me a hideous case of the creeps.

A trifle less subtle than the Crow was a visitor to B-3, the primary habitat of the L.O.J.L.'s. One evening I was sitting in the doctors' dining room when I heard a stat page for me come over the loudspeaker. The word stat is an abbreviation of the Latin *statim*, meaning "at once." Thus it signifies an emergency, and when you get a stat page, you don't bother to answer it by phone— you just get your ass to your ward posthaste. You may have to resuscitate a patient, or contend with a similar catastrophe.

Swallowing a mouthful of spaghetti, I took the three flights of stairs two steps at a time and charged down the corridor. Even before I turned the corner, I could hear a fearsome commotion. It sounded as though there was a riot on my ward.

Arriving at the entry to B-3, I found that to be literally the case. The place was in an unparalleled (even for The Vue) turmoil. At first glance, it looked as though every lady on the ward who was not totally bedridden was on her feet in the middle of the room— hitting, clawing, biting, and screeching at an old man who was ineffectually trying to defend himself. As one of the ladies spat directly into his face, another let loose a bone-shatterer of a kick directly to the shin. The old man unleashed a blood-curdling howl and began to sink slowly into the west.

"What the hell's happening here?" I hollered. Remembering Mr. Harris' prostitute, I wondered whether this was a dirty old man who had tried a similar practice in reverse. So to speak.

Both the nurse and the aide shrugged. They had seen the man come onto the ward, but had just assumed he was somebody's visitor. He had, however, proceeded directly to the center of the ward, from which point he had announced that the Jews were a race accursed, one inevitably doomed to spend all eternity in a warm, humid, sulfurous locale other than New York City. Therefore, by the power somehow or other vested in him by the Lord Himself, he had come to offer salvation to the Jews via the mechanism of conversion.

It was then that I realized that all the rioting females were L.O.J.L.'s. The gentile patients were still in their beds.

Apparently, at first, the L.O.J.L.'s had been mildly amused by their would-be Savior's offer. However, when no one came forth to take the cure, the man became impatient and began to berate his Semitic audience for their stiff necks and foolhardy pride. At that point, all traces of tolerance vanished, and the nurse and the aide realized that mutiny was in the air.

The preacher man looked around him. In those days, the name cards on the foot of each bed were color-coded according to the religion of the patient. Blue was the Jewish color. The eyes of the Right Hand of the Lord fell on the combination he had been looking for: a blue card and an unconscious lady. He moved with alacrity to Sarah Goldkin's bedside.

Mrs. Goldkin had been felled by a stroke a few weeks previously. She hadn't moved since, and furthermore, she would not move again until the sound of Gabriel's trumpet echoed through the boondocks. The man licked his chops and announced her salvation to the residents of B-3. This set off a buzz of angry muttering, and the nurse moved to get rid of the guy. Before she could, though, he sprinkled Mrs. Goldkin with some water from a container he pulled from his pocket. With that, all hell broke loose.

The majority of the old women on B-3 had emigrated to America as girls or young women in order to escape the anti-Semitic pogroms of eastern Europe. On the Lower East Side of New York, they had found freedom from fear, which all their lives had remained their most precious possession. Now, the sight of this *meshuggener*, this crazy *goy*, trying to separate their helpless sister from her faith, aroused in them all the fear and hostility that had lain latent all these years. In a body, they attacked.

I looked the situation over and decided that if I waited to call the guards, the angry old Jewish ladies might well have their victim dismembered before the militia could arrive. It was obvious that prompt and direct action would be necessary.

I plunged into the action and snaked my way toward the center of the furious *yentes*. As I had hoped, the sight of my white coat and pants cooled them off sufficiently for me to be able to drag the scuffed sidewalk preacher out of their midst and to the front of the ward. As we neared the entryway to the corridor, he scrambled to his feet and wrenched free from my grip. Then he turned to face the crowd of women still standing in the middle of the ward.

All pretense of religiosity had left him, and the pure hatred of the frustrated bigot blazed from his eyes. "Kikes!" he screamed at the top of his lungs. "Mockies! Dirty, lousy sheeny bastards! You'll all go right straight to hell, 'n' you kin see if I'll care. Serve y'all right, too."

I got hold of the man's elbow with one hand and his collar with the other, led him to the elevator, put him on, and advised him that it might be better in the future were he to confine his activities to street corners. So much for the Lost Souls of Bellevue.

I thought that was the end of the episode, but I was very wrong. Upon my return to the ward, the entire body of L.O.J.L.'s met me at the doorway. Literally wailing, they were pulling their hair and gnashing their teeth. At first I couldn't figure out for the life of me what was upsetting them so, but finally, the more-nearly composed of them led me to understand that they were concerned for Mrs. Goldkin's well-being in the afterlife, should she die a *goy*. It helped not in the least to explain that Mrs. Goldkin hadn't accepted the unwelcome sacraments, that, in fact, she probably hadn't even been aware they were being offered her. The only thing that mattered to her wardmates was that, willing or not, she had been baptized. In the end, we had to call a rabbi up to the ward; he conducted the proper decontamination ceremony and the other patients went back to their beds content. A few days later, Mrs. Goldkin went to her rest, secure in the faith of her ancestors.

Undoubtedly the most embarrassing experience I ever had with a Bellevue visitor was the time I played host to Dr. Burleigh-Toft. It happened one November night during my stint as a gynecology resident.

About seven o'clock in the evening, as I was sitting in the gynecology examining area, waiting for the inevitable flood of referrals from the Admitting Office, in walked a man dressed in an expensive gray woolen suit. At The Vue, this in itself would have been sufficient to attract attention, but in addition he was wearing a dark bowler hat and sported an impressive waxed mustache. Without the least hesitation, he walked up to the desk, extended his hand in greeting, and said, "Dr. Karp?"

I acknowledged that that was indeed my name.

"Ah, delighted," said the man, removing his hat and placing it on the desk in front of me. "They told me I'd find you here. My name is Burleigh-Toft—Dr. Charles Burleigh-Toft. I'm a gynecologist from Liverpool, England. I'm touring the States, and am to give a talk to your group tomorrow about the bacteriology of pelvic infections in Great Britain. But since I've nothing particular to do this evening, I thought I might drop by and just visit informally a bit. You know, Bellevue Hospital is famous 'round the world, and I've always wished for the opportunity to see it in action, as you might say. Wouldja mind terribly if I were to tag along with you as you do your work?"

Dr. Burleigh-Toft's voice absolutely dripped London fog. Would I mind if he were to watch me work a bit? I was flattered silly. It was heady stuff for a mere first-year resident to be asked to provide the evening's entertainment for a visiting fireman. I told the doctor that it would be my pleasure.

Since nothing was happening at the moment, he pulled up a chair and began to ask me questions about the sorts of patients we were accustomed to treating at The Vue. I was in the middle of telling him about the grisliest of our cases of infected abortion when the aide from the A.O. wheeled in a young woman who was arranged in a side saddle position in a wheelchair.

The nurse came from the ward to help, and I introduced Dr. Burleigh-Toft to her. Then she put the patient up for examination. As my British visitor and I walked into the examining cubicle, the reason for the lady's peculiar posture in the wheelchair became painfully obvious. She was suffering from a Bartholin-duct abscess, a type of boil on the vulva. I whistled.

"I say, that *is* a nahsty one," said Dr. Burleigh-Toft.

I ordered a sedative for the patient, and then, using every ounce of ham in me, I demonstrated my magnificent technique of incision and drainage. The Englishman watched closely over my left shoulder.

"That should make her more comfortable," I said.

"Oh, indeed," said Dr. Burleigh-Toft. "Very nicely done. Very nice."

The next patient to come in had a pelvic infection. Since this was Dr. Burleigh-Toft's area of special expertise, I was delighted to have him examine her with me. He performed an extremely long and careful pelvic evaluation, during which he wrinkled and unwrinkled his brow several times. Then he asked me whether I had noticed the thickening at the sides of the uterus.

"No," I said. "Honestly, I can't really say I did."

"Gonorrhea," said Dr. Burleigh-Toft. "When you feel thickening around the uterus, you know it's gonorrhea. Other bacteria don't cause that."

"I don't remember seeing that in any of my textbooks," I blurted out, and immediately wanted to gnaw furrows in my tongue.

Fortunately, my foreign visitor didn't appear to be insulted. He laughed lightly. "Quite right," he said. "It's not in any text. But I've noticed it repeatedly over the years, and I've really very little doubt that it will one day be accepted as a standard diagnostic sign."

I gratefully let the matter drop, and we went on to examine the next patient, an older woman with a prolapsed uterus. After that, we helped a patient complete her miscarriage. It turned into a busy night, and Dr. Burleigh-Toft followed me from cubicle to cubicle, watching interestedly, and now and then offering a comment. More than once, I remarked to myself how nice it was to see someone who had been able to maintain such obvious enthusiasm for his work.

About ten o'clock, Dr. Burleigh-Toft glanced at his watch. "As much as I hate to, I think I really must be going," he said. "But I've had a *most* enjoyable evening, and I thank you. And by the way, I shall certainly commend you to your chairman tomorrow."

That reminded me. "What time is your talk?" I asked him. "I wouldn't want to miss it."

He shook his head. "I'm not quite certain," he said. "Sometime in the morning. I expect they'll announce it over the 'speaker." We shook hands, he gave me a hearty slap on the arm, and went out the door.

Morning came and went, but there was no loudspeaker announcement. Nor was there any break in the usual work routine. I began to feel some nasty vibes. At lunch, I casually asked the senior resident at what time Dr. Burleigh-Toft was scheduled to speak.

"Who?" he asked, without much interest.

"Dr. Burleigh-Toft," I said. "From Liverpool. I thought he was scheduled to give a lecture today on pelvic infections."

"Never heard of him," said the senior resident.

"Oh," I said. "Isn't he visiting the department?"

"I've never heard of any gynecologist named Burleigh-Toft," said the senior. "And I know there're no departmental visitors right now. In fact, there haven't been any for weeks. Where'd you get that idea from?"

"One of the interns mentioned it to me," I said, and quickly changed the subject to our surgical case of that day. I may have been stupid, but I wasn't dumb enough to tell the senior resident that I had given the world's champion Peeping Tom the greatest keyhole he'd ever had.

16

A Blood Brotherhood

Traditionally, the stepchild of every hospital in the world, Bellevue included, has been its blood bank. This is the perpetual crisis spot, always hanging on at best by a slender red thread. Then, every so often, some guy will come wheeling into the Emergency Room, shot through the liver or the spleen. Before he finally dies, he'll receive thirty or forty transfusions, thereby causing the blood bank to suffer a shortage of blood as severe as his own. As a result, everyone starts screaming, a drive is hastily mounted, and the deficit restored before the supply runs totally dry.

At that point, with his blood pressure a few points higher and the lining of his stomach a few microns thinner, the director of the blood bank goes wild and makes pronouncements. He cancels elective surgery for patients without blood donors. Emergency cases who require transfusions are hounded, along with their relatives. Some especially astute hospitals, understanding full well the road to an intern's heart, recompense each house officer fifty cents or a dollar for every donor he sends to the bank. These few institutions, may I add, rarely have blood bank difficulties. Anemic visitors, yes. But anemic blood banks, no.

However, in most hospitals, it's all over in a week or so. The blood bank director takes his tranquilizers, the rules get stretched to the point where they finally rupture, and everyone goes back to S.O.P. until the next nightmarish Emergency Room crisis.

The director of the Bellevue Hospital blood bank in the early 1960's was Dr. Arthur R. Stephenson, a renowned hematologist. He was a tall, spare man with the stooped shoulders that come from thirty years of staring down into microscopes, and a countenance which one would expect on someone with a duodenal ulcer or perhaps bad hemorrhoids. The man appeared to be perpetually in pain. Which he may well have been. The directorship of the Bellevue blood bank was a job I wouldn't have wished on my worst enemy. Out of sheer pity, we always tried to get Dr. Stephenson and his workers as many donors as we could.

One day, however, the chief resident of obstetrics and gynecology called me up and told me that our blood replacement efforts were not up to snuff.

"What do you mean?" I asked him. "Last month our service got three more donors than we used transfusions. You know we work at it. Why doesn't the blood bank beat on the surgeons—they were short 156 pints last month?"

"I guess Stephenson figures why should he knock himself out on guys who won't put out anyway?" answered the C.R. "He probably thinks if he puts the screws to us, there's at least a chance he'll get some bottles of blood out of it." The chief paused a minute, but before I could say anything, he added, "And if he doesn't get blood, he's going to cancel all our elective surgery. And the surgeons', too, by the way. So, if you and the other guys don't get with it in a hurry, your chief won't have anything to do all day but beat on you and make your life miserable. 'Bye, Lar, ol' buddy."

I couldn't really get mad. I knew Dr. Stephenson must have been up tight against the wall, and as blood bank director, a man is more than entitled to periodic bouts of rational irrationality. I sat down for a few minutes and pondered the situation.

Now there existed a custom at The Vue whereby every woman who delivered a baby there was supposed to have two persons donate blood for her. This was a difficult rule to enforce: after all, one can't hold a baby back until the mother has coughed up her two pints of blood. So a few of the women sent in a husband and a brother, a larger number got one donor, but most would provide none. A surprising number of these welfare patients' husbands offered to pay for the blood. They'd just shrug when we told them that you can't transfuse a dollar bill to a dying patient. One day, I asked one of the Puerto Rican nurses' aides why the resistance. She told me that Latin men believed that donating blood drains off their virility and robs them of their potency. She giggled.

"What's so funny?" I asked.

"I wuz jes' t'inkin, Dr. Karp," she said. "Maybe you could git *my* husbin' to give some blood sometimes."

I directed my thoughts back to the major problem at hand, and decided that the only thing to do was to enforce the law. So I got together with the rest of the residents and the medical students, and we agreed that no patient would be discharged until she had arranged for her blood donations.

As the maternity ward began to fill up, and as large numbers of men began to consider the thought of cooking and cleaning *ad infinitum,* they made their way to the blood bank, bringing back their donation receipts to exchange for their wives. Of course, there were the imaginative fellows like the two-hundred-pound mesomorph who sought me out to explain that as much as he'd have liked to help me out, he simply couldn't, because he had anemia—"real bad anemia." I told him to go down to the blood bank anyway, that not only would they not let him give blood if he were anemic, but they'd see he got proper treatment for his condition.

"And if I am anemic, Doc, then can I take my wife home?"

"Then," I said, "you can get your brother in. Or your sister. Or your father. Or anyone in your family who isn't anemic." The guy trudged downstairs, was relieved of a pint of virility and potency, and took home his wife.

This went on for two weeks. Great hordes of friends and relatives of parturient women flocked to the blood bank. Then one day I looked at the report, and did a double take. I couldn't believe it. Perhaps for the first time in history, the Bellevue Hospital blood bank was in the black. I picked up the phone and called the bank. One of the assistant directors answered, and he was euphoric. "I don't know what the hell you're doing over there," he burbled, "but keep it up."

I told the guy what we were doing over there. He whistled. "Gaaah-damn!" he yelled. "That is just great. Really great. Keep it up, now, you understand?"

We kept it up for another few days. At that juncture, I received a phone call from Mr. Wilson, who was one of the hospital administrators. Mr. Wilson wanted to know what was all this about holding patients prisoner on the maternity ward.

"Why, Mr. Wilson," I said. "Whatever in the world can you be talking about?"

I heard Mr. Wilson choke a little on the other end, and I felt a brief twinge of conscience. Mr. W. was really a very nice fellow. But business is business. So I just sat there and waited.

"I got a call from the employer of one of your patients," he finally said, in tight, clipped words. "He told me that the lady had told him she was being 'held' at the hospital for lack of blood donors."

Such episodes help to clarify the basis for our acts of humanity. The efficiency of this guy's factory had probably been lowered by a factor of one cog's worth.

"Mr. Wilson," I said. "You know that every obstetrical patient is supposed to donate two pints of blood, and she hasn't."

Mr. W. was beginning to get angry. "Well, you let her go anyway."

"I can't do that," I said. "Dr. Stephenson's crew feels that it's necessary to get every blood donor we possibly can. So all our residents have agreed to enforce the two-donors-per-patient rule. If you call our chief resident and he says it's okay, I'll discharge the patient."

Mr. Wilson's teeth ground audibly, and he said he'd do that. I thanked him, and went back to work.

A short while later I got a call from the chief. Mr. Wilson had called him, as well as the blood bank A.D. who was on duty at that moment. The chief resident advised me that everyone else concerned had concluded that it would be best were we to yield on the matter. "We've made our point," he said. "Now, if the administrator wants us to send the patient home, I think we should." He chuckled. "You did good." I smiled, hung up, and called Mr. Wilson back.

The administrator sounded a bit calmer now. He explained that the blood bank official had led him to understand the full state of affairs, as had the chief resident. "But," he went on, "we really can't hold patients prisoners, you know. They could sue us."

"We haven't held anyone prisoner," I said. "We just haven't discharged them. If they've wanted to leave the hospital, we haven't interfered with them in any way. In fact, we didn't even threaten to refuse them follow-up care."

Mr. Wilson uh-hummed for a couple of seconds, and then asked, "How about this particular woman? Did she actually receive any blood?"

"Only four pints," I answered. "She had a post-partum hemorrhage."

"Well," said Mr. Wilson. "Isn't that interesting? I think I'll call her boss and tell him that. In fact, I'll tell him the whole situation."

"That sounds good," I said. I got ready to go back to work.

"But we'll just have to stop enforcing that rule," went on Mr. Wilson. "You've seen those newspaper guys who're always going up and down the corridors, trying to smell out a good scandal or two. Just think what one of them could make out of this business, if he got onto it."

And so, the Bellevue blood bank situation returned to normal. Dr. Stephenson and his gallant crew continued to beat their heads against the wall, trying to keep the stores in the blood bank one step above disaster level. When things got bad enough, another drive was organized, everyone congratulated himself, and then it was downhill again for another few months. The crises went round and round. Every so often, some poor guy bled to death while a frantic effort was being made to locate enough of the proper type of blood for him. Eventually this sort of tragedy happened several times too often, and blood banks began to centralize their facilities and their resources, to provide greater cushions against sudden large demands on their reserves. This expedient has helped to some degree, of course, but it's not nearly a satisfactory solution. Nor can such really be expected to be found, as long as we continue to show great concern for the efficient functioning of our factories and for what the newspapers may say about us, while demonstrating much less anxiety about safeguarding the lives of our neighbors, our families, and even ourselves.

17

They Shall Beat
the Interns into
Pruning Hooks

In a place like The Vue, you might expect that there would be a
good deal of violence. Actually, there was relatively little of an
obvious sort. Bellevue was years ahead in pioneering the "better
latent than blatant" theory. Although there was constant friction
among doctors, administrators, nurses, aides, ancillary help, and
patients, rarely did it erupt into a good, healthy fracas. Like the
rest of Bellevue, it just festered quietly. Periodically, it would
burst out here or there; then the troops would clean up the mess
and, for a while longer, business would go on as usual.

The persons responsible for keeping the peace in The Vue
were the guards, an elite corps of ex-cops and would-be cops
employed for the purpose by the City of New York. They were
directed to trouble spots by the paging operators.

The paging system at Bellevue was truly gothic. Twenty-four
hours a day the loudspeakers would blare forth with requests for
doctors to call their wards. The speakers were never muted at
night, and I never could see how any of the patients ever managed
to get a night's sleep. The operators themselves were a riot. Only
those with the thickest New York accents and the most outlandish
Bronx twangs were chosen. When my friend Dr. Dahl was needed,
it was, "Dokta Dawl, Dokta Daviddawl, Dokta Dawl, Dokta
Daviddawl." Once was never enough. And when we heard, in
singsong tones, "Pagin' d' gahds, d' gahds, d' gahds! Pagin' d'
gahds, d' gahds, d' gahds!" we knew that, somewhere in the
hospital, brains were being spilled on the concrete floors, or were

about to be. Then we'd see d' gahds, nightsticks in hand, charging through the corridors. We'd head the other way.

When I was a medical student, one of my interns was Frank Melnor. At the time, Frank was working on the neurology ward. Many neurology patients were sad cases, who, as the result of brain injury or stroke, were totally unconscious and would remain so until the day they would die, a time which the physicians were morally bound to defer as long as possible.

One night, Frank Melnor decided that one of his unresponsive patients had pneumonia and needed a chest X-ray. He wanted to put the patient onto a stretcher and wheel him to the radiology department. The trouble was, this particular man weighed more than two hundred pounds. So Frank went into the ward office to look for help. An aide was sitting there reading a comic book, and Frank requested that he stop long enough to help lift the patient onto the stretcher.

Since the aide didn't budge, Frank thought he might not have heard the request, so he repeated it in a louder voice. However, this also brought no response.

Now Frank decided that he was being ignored, so he hollered at the aide to quit fooling aroung and lend a hand immediately. When the aide remained immobile, Frank could stand no more, so he ran over, ripped the comic book out of the aide's hands, and flung it across the room.

This was a foolish move, because the aide looked like the late Sonny Liston in his prime. Very slowly he rose to his feet, and very slowly he advanced on Frank. Grabbing the intern by his lapels, he raised Frank off the floor and, in a monotonic drawl, patiently informed him that another such performance would certainly be Frank's last. Then he let go, picked up his comic book, and went back to his reading.

That was not the end, though. The next day the aide reported Frank to his union leader, who in turn saw to it that Frank was reprimanded by the hospital administrator for attempting to use physical force on the aide. The fact that the aide had considered it appropriate to sit and read a comic book for eight hours between punching in and out was of no import. It was like the time that one of the interns, while wheeling his patient to the X-ray department, was thrown off an elevator to make room for the elevator operator's friend, the garbage man with his sacks of goodies. The next morning, when the intern complained to an administrator, he was told to shut up and get back to work. "I can always get another intern," said the administrator. "But I can't get another elevator operator." That wasn't really true, of course. But the interns weren't unionized and the elevator operators were. In any event, Frank Melnor had to solve his personnel problem by getting a portable X-ray on his patient.

Sometimes one of the members of the Bellevue animal population would figure in an episode of violence. You have to remember that since it was located on the banks of the East River, The Vue was home to a very large number of very large beasts. Gigantic rats, mice, and roaches wandered fearlessly through the corridors. They were part of the Bellevue folklore. For example, rumor had it that an intern, while carrying a blood specimen through the basement passageway to the pathology building, was devoured by an alligator that had taken up residence in the huge water puddles on the floors. Then there was the story of the intern who had been run down and killed in the parking lot by a Volkswagen. When the witnesses chased down the vehicle and brought it to a halt, they found that it was really just a cockroach. I don't believe the story, though. No one in New York would bother to chase down a hit-and-run cockroach.

Cockroach stories sometimes crossed the line into the real world. It was nothing short of nauseating, after having washed off a lady who was about to deliver a baby, to see a large roach crawl out from beneath the sterile sheets and onto her belly. The lady was never terribly happy about it either. Then there was the time that one of the residents bit into a meatball in the dining room and uncovered one of the little beasties. A number of us at the table turned pale, but the unlucky fellow didn't bat an eye. He just picked up his plate and carried it into the kitchen where Miz Matthews, the dietitian, was standing. Showing her the evidence, he said, "Miz Matthews, you know, you really ought to serve the cockroaches on separate platters."

The most ubiquitous vermin were the mice. As soon as the lights were turned out at eleven o'clock, the Grand Army of the Republic began its nightly march. You could hear them scampering across the floor until morning. They ate any food that happened to be left out by an unwary patient. In fact, sometimes they ate the patients. They really did. We had to be certain that the moribund and the helpless were kept near the front of the ward, where the occasional activity and the light from the nurses' desk would keep the patients from being devoured by the gang of hungry little omnivores. The Bowery Bums knew all this very well, and when they were admitted, they'd plead for a bed near the front.

The hatred of the bums for the mice was epic. One particular fellow harbored an especial loathing for the beasts, and as he became stronger and consequently was moved progressively farther to the back, his anger became more and more vocal. The end, as far as he was concerned, came one night when one of the Rodent Raiders not only had the temerity to make off with the chunk of cake he had left on his nighttable, but actually made his getaway across the sleeping man's face and then down the bedclothes. By the time we made rounds the next morning, our livid patient informed us that that was the absolute end, that he had not the least intention of putting up with any more murine indignities. We shrugged and went on the the next bed. Any attempt to rid Bellevue Hospital of mice would have been comparable in effect to emptying one's bladder into the Pacific Ocean.

That night, my friend Harvey Brown was working on that ward. Harvey was a good-natured ectomorph who maintained his skinny habitus by constantly worrying about what misfortune was going to befall him next. Harvey went through life dreading the adversities that he was certain were in store for him, and when they did come, he lavished all his love and attention on them. This being the case, you may be certain that the night something bizarre happened, Harvey Brown would be there to enter fully into the experience.

This particular night, it happened to be pretty quiet, so not quite believing his good fortune, Harvey put his head down on the nurses' desk and went to sleep. It was 2 A.M. He hadn't slept long when he was awakened by a tremendous clatter. Harvey leaped from his chair, certain that the old building was falling down around him. Flicking on the ward lights as he came down, he heard a raucous, "Hah! Take that, yuh sonavabitch. I gotcha!" The Lord never saithed "Vengeance is mine" with more feeling. Harvey looked toward the back of the ward, where the vengeful one sat triumphantly in bed. Five yards away lay the bloody corpse of a fat gray mouse, the remains of a candy bar lying just beyond its paws, the whole scene representing a living (in a sense) testimonial to the fact that excess weight is bad for your health. The lethal weapon lay where it had bounced and finally come to rest, all the way across the ward. The patient then proudly told Harvey the story of how he had left the piece of candy bar on the nighttable, and then had sat up, motionless, for three hours. When the thief had appeared and then had made off with the goodies, his malefactor—on the run and in the dark, may I remind you—cold-cocked him and laid him low with a bull's-eye pitch of his metal bedside urinal. This having happened in 1962, I wondered what the New York Mets would have given to have had this guy on their mound staff.

From time to time, other patients provided a little violent diversion. One night during the year I was a resident in gynecology, I was taking a history from a patient. She was a fortyish, fattish little lady with pale reddish hair and a pale whitish face. She was to undergo a hysterectomy and bladder repair. After I had gone through all the details of her incontinent behavior, I proceeded on to the general medical history. This is an assortment of questions which patients often find irrelevant and unrelated to their problems. Sometimes they're right. We like to think we're checking for previously unrecognized conditions that would, for instance, make the proposed surgery needlessly hazardous. I questioned the woman as to her previous illnesses and operations. Then I checked into the possibilities of heart or lung diseases. All answers were negative. The patient assured me that she felt just fine. She was most congenial, and we were having a nice talk. Then I got to the gastrointestinal system. "Do you have any trouble with your bowel movements?" I asked.

The woman paused and thought for a moment. "Well, Doc," she said, "Only thing 'at bothers me at all is them green worms."

This only took me back a little bit. I figured that she happened to have some pinworms. Pinworms, however, are not green, and I so informed her.

"Oh no," she said. "These worms are green. Little and green. And they're always crawling out of my rectum." She looked intently at me and I began to feel a little uneasy. My God, what kind of intestinal parasites could these be? I asked the patient whether she had any idea as to how the green worms had come to take up residence in her nether regions, at the same time thinking that it would be a cold day in hell before I'd ever do a pelvic examination on her.

The woman seemed exasperated by my question. She put her hands on her hips and gave me a quizzical look. My discomfort mounted. "Well, Doc," she said, "they're not only down there."

"Where else are they?" I faltered.

Now she began to get excited. "When I brush my teeth, they crawl out between my teeth and my gums. And then when I clean out my ears, they crawl out from there."

Now I was beginning to get the message. This was a case for the boys with the white coats and the butterfly nets. I motioned to the nurse who was standing nearby, taking in the scene with wide eyes and mouth. She quietly moved to the phone and put in a call to the hatch.

This was a very good thing to have done, because now, suddenly, there was no holding down our patient. She was up on her feet, hair flying, eyes bright and glazed, and arms flapping. She began to scream at the top of her lungs, "And that's not all—they're all over my apartment. They come out of the water taps when I turn them on. They crawl around on the walls. They come in under the doors." She turned and looked into my eyes. "I can't get rid of them, do you hear me, I can't get rid of them no matter what I do."

It was really the most amazing transformation I've ever seen. From a pleasant, apparently rational woman to an out-and-out raging lunatic in all of three minutes. I tried to calm her down by changing the subject, but she'd have none of that ploy. She ranted on and on about the green worms, how she figured that her husband had planted them on her before he had left, and how she couldn't rid herself of them.

At this point in walked the two psych attendants with a wheelchair and a strait jacket. My patient took one look at them, recognition dawned, and then she looked back at me. "You son-of-a-bitch," she screamed. "You dirty, no-good son-of-a-bitch." She lunged across the desk at me. The attendants grabbed her as I dove under the desk.

You can't imagine how that woman fought. While she held off two burly psych-ward attendants, she still had strength enough to call me names I blush to remember, let alone repeat. Finally the nurse had to call for two of d' gahds to come up and help get her restrained before she killed the attendants. At length they got her strait-jacketed into the wheelchair, and the four of them wheeled her off down that long, dark corridor to the hatch. I could hear her yelling and the wheelchair bouncing all the way down the hall.

The chief resident was a bit unhappy the next morning when he found that his hysterectomy had vaporized. When he heard the story of the night before, he gave me the fish eye.

"Go on down to the hatch and operate on her if you want," I said. "Just don't blame me when you come back covered with green worms that you can't get rid of." He wandered off, muttering about the impossibility of running a service where the residents were nuttier than the patients. I didn't see him again all day.

Another memorable violent patient was the J-O Lady. J-O Rat Paste was a commonly used pesticide in some New York homes. Among our Puerto Rican clientele, it also served another function. They used it for suicide attempts. They spread it on bread and ate it as sandwiches. I'm not kidding; they really did. The active ingredient was white phosphorus, a lethal liver and kidney poison which takes about a week to reduce these organs to functionless masses of pulp. Hence, attempts at suicide with J-O were uniformly successful. This was really very sad, because most of these suicide attempts were just gestures, employed to frighten a husband, lover, son, or parent.

The J-O Lady came in one Friday night. In a fit of pique against her boyfriend, she had dissolved her rat paste in a glass of orange juice and swigged it down. Later on, when we asked her why she had chosen this method (she freely admitted she had done it "just to teach my boyfriend a lesson"), she said it was because that was what her sister had used to do away with herself (for a similar reason) three years previously. You go figure it out.

In any case, when the J-O Lady came in, she was in no mood to be cooperative. When I approached her to try to empty her stomach, she spat in my face. Let me tell you, phosphorescent spit burns. To evacuate her stomach contents we used a wide, red rubber tube whose real name was the Ewald tube. It was popularly known as the Garden Hose. She took one look at that and clawed my hand, leaving five red tracks.

At this juncture I figured I'd better call in the reserves. An explanation by a Spanish-speaking aide got the aide a faceful of phosphorus-laden saliva. So we resorted to finesse. Two two-hundred-pound female Emergency Room aides, known as the Bookends, sat on the patient and restrained her arms and legs while I slipped the Garden Hose down her gullet.

As the tube hit the stomach, thick white fumes began to come out from it. It was as though the woman's stomach were on fire. In fact, it may have been. The more she struggled, the thicker came the fumes. We tried to pass materials down the tube that might have neutralized the phosphorus before it could be absorbed into her body, but the fumes only came thicker and faster. Then I began to notice that the fumes had a particularly acrid character. Still, they issued forth.

Of course, none of our work did any good, and the woman died ten days later, yellow all over and not producing any urine. She turned out to be a very nice person, and we all felt very unhappy as we watched her die. Her boyfriend allowed as how he had been taught a good lesson, but he claimed not to have been able to figure out the reason for the whole thing.

As for me, I woke up the morning after having lavaged the stomach of the J-O Lady and coughed. It felt as though my entire chest were on fire. Then I tried to call down by phone to the ward and discovered that I couldn't talk. Since I never had had bronchitis or laryngitis before, this all struck me as odd. Then I remembered the smoke of the night before. That was it: I had a beautiful case of chemical bronchitis. Those phosphorus fumes must have done some job on my windpipes. Every winter, now, almost as soon as I catch a cold, I become voiceless. I guess I'll carry my souvenir of Bellevue for some time to come. My wife tells me I shouldn't complain, that I might have caught syphilis. The logic of the argument leaves something to be desired, but the sentiment is unmistakable.

Not only the patients caused violence on the wards. Sometimes their relatives did. New York has always been the nation's leader in style-setting and, as such, long before race riots had become a national way of life, it was not uncommon for an intern in the middle of examining a Negro patient to be interrupted by an angry relative warning that the patient had certainly better improve forthwith if the doctor knew what was good for him, and that the era of white doctors giving short shrift to black patients was now over. One night in the Emergency Room, I was sewing up a laceration on a black woman's scalp when suddenly the door to the room burst open, and in ran the patient's boyfriend. "Git yo' god-damn white han's offa her," he shrieked. "I wan' a *black* doctuh t' take care a her. No white doctuh's good enough t' take care a her, y' unnerstan'?"

I moved to get out of the room while my epidermis was still intact when the lady let loose at her boyfriend with, "You shut up you' mouf! Dis doctuh's sewin' up mah haid real nice wif his white han's, an' it don't even hurt none. So if you don't shut up you' black mouf, ah'll turn it red fo' you." With this, the young militant sagged his way back out the door, looking about half as big as when he had come in. Thanking God that there was a back door to the treatment room that I could use later, I finished the job quickly and quietly.

The most outlandish story of violent relatives involved the time that a gypsy queen suffered an attack of heart failure in the neighborhood and her followers brought her to The Vue. The internists checked her out and discovered that she had rheumatic heart disease and that she would need surgery to open one of the valves so that the blood might pass through unimpeded. So she was transferred to surgery and the operation was scheduled.

Meanwhile the entire caravan set up encampment on the front lawn (such as it was) of the hospital. Shortly thereafter, a story began to circulate through The Vue. Supposedly, a couple of d' gahds, noticing the gypsies' infringement, had sauntered out to request that the troops vacate. The gypsies listened politely; when the speech was finished, two of the young gypsies held knives to the throats of d' gahds while other gypsies held them immobile and incommunicado. Upon being released a few mintues later, the guards decided it would be only humane to permit the poor people to remain on the premises.

And so, in any case, they stayed. Somehow or other, these illiterate nomads were able to pick out on sight all the many doctors who had seen to the health and well-being of their queen. Furthermore, whenever any of the doctors entered or left the building, he'd be greeted by one of the men, who would say, "Gypsy Queen die, doctor die." Then he'd make a slashing motion across his throat with his knife blade.

The doctors found this behavior disconcerting, especially when they considered that a middle-aged woman undergoing heart surgery is not exactly an insurance salesman's dream. So they began to try to leave the building via alternate doors. No dice. It took the gypsies one day to figure out they were being evaded. From that point, they began to post guards at each doorway. What's more, they didn't distinguish among internists, surgeons, and medical students. Any guy in a white suit who had examined the queen was given full coverage. Needless to say, this became a bit nerve-racking.

Finally one of my friends who was an intern on the ward figured out what to do. By going up the inside stairway and across the roof, he could cut down a corridor into the kitchen and sneak out the delivery door that was used for food and garbage. He was also smart enough not to tell anyone else involved about his technique; the gypsies seemed not to miss just one doctor. This whole thing went on for six weeks, until the Queen of the Gypsies, her cardiac pathways having been successfully Roto-Rootered, was discharged from the hospital. Then the caravan packed up and left, never to be seen again.

When the navy drafted me and sent me from Bellevue to Quonset Point, Rhode Island, I took a look around me at the peaceful countryside and decided I had been fortunate to escape in one piece from New York.

Then, not three months after I had gone to Rhode Island, I noticed an article in the Providence paper which mentioned that a resident at New York's Bellevue Hospital had been shot. As I read on, I discovered that he had been a first-year resident in obstetrics, and that he had been plugged while on the maternity ward during visiting hours the night before. He was described as a hero: he had seen a man pull a gun on his wife and had stepped between the couple and tried to break it up. Whereupon the husband had opened fire on the would-be peacemaker, damaging his lung and pulmonary vein. At that point, the guards came on the scene, disarmed that attacker, and rushed the resident to the surgery suite. The article stated that the surgeons had sewed up his supernumerary orifices, and that now, forty-six blood transfusions later, they held out some hope that he might just possibly recover.

I put down the paper and looked at my wife, who had been reading the article with me. "What would you have done if that'd happened to you last year?" she asked.

I pride myself on being a basically honest man. Cowardly, but honest. "I would have run as fast as I could," I said, "and hid behind the nearest piece of metal."

We followed the recovery of the resident in the newspapers and by notes to and from my friends at The Vue. It drove me wild: I couldn't figure out what had ever possessed the resident to try to disarm an angry Bellevue husband. No self-respecting New Yorker I had known at Bellevue would have even thought of doing such a thing. I figured the guy must have been a Midwesterner, newly arrived at The Vue for his training and not yet accustomed to the prevailing New York mentality, which dictates that one watches placidly while women are shot, stabbed, raped, and/or dismembered. What can you expect from a greenhorn?

Six months passed. The resident finally recovered sufficiently to return to work, and my wife and I took a trip to New York. I went over to The Vue and visited with my old friends. While we were talking, a pale, fragile-looking fellow walked up and joined the group. One of my friends introduced me to him; I immediately recognized his name. "You're the resident who got shot," I said. Before he could squirm uncomfortably, I added, "Where are you from?"

"New York," he answered quietly, his eyes looking mildly at me from behind his horn rims. "Why?"

"Because I can't figure out what in God's name ever possessed you to place your one and only body between that woman and her husband," I said.

Now he looked uncomfortable. "Oh God," he said. "Did you read that in the papers?"

"Sure," I said. "I just couldn't believe that you tried to take the gun away from that guy."

"Nuts," said the resident. "I didn't step between them. And I certainly didn't try to take the gun away."

Now I was puzzled. But he continued: "Actually, what happened was, I was running away; I was trying to get behind the metal wall in the Examining Room. The guy's first shot went through a nurse's cap and the next one got me."

"But the newspapers said—"

"I don't care what they said. I guess they wrote it up that way because it was a better story. I mean, how would it sound if they tried to sell newspapers that said, Fleeing resident shot by husband with lousy aim'?" He laughed. "He shot me in the back, you know."

Well, I only know what I read in the papers.

18

And Gladly Did They Learn

Everybody has his own idea as to what a medical student is like. Some say he's a clean-shaven young man with determined bloodshot eyes who sits at the kitchen table studying until 2 A.M. His wife after an evening of being dutifully quiet, slumbers alone in the bedroom while a torn window shade does a poor job of keeping out the light from the street lamp strategically placed right outside the tenement window. Other people believe him to be an ever-jolly soul who divides his time between dropping stolen cadaver penises on crowded buses and deflowering panting, big-breasted student nurses. More recently he may be seen as a frustrated social worker who cuts out of his neurology lectures and refuses to learn gross anatomy, the better to spend his time tilting at the A.M.A., going to the storefront clinic in the ghetto where he dispenses what he figures is good medical advice, or doing other meaningful and relevant things.

Whatever medical students really are like, though, I think it can truthfully be said that they are also often quite funny. Not because of any intrinsic humorous propensity particular to the type, but because of the situation in which they are placed. They're funny in the same way your teen-aged daughter is funny when she flounces around the dining room in her first bra. It's interesting to watch someone's reactions when he finally finds himself eating with the grownups.

During my second year at medical school I got to put on a white coat for the first time. I stood in front of the mirror in my room for a full twenty minutes. I looked at myself with the buttons both open and closed. I looked at profiles and frontal views. I tried on three different ties. Finally ready, I went across the street to the hospital for the ophthalmology lesson. With my shiny new ophthalmoscope, I spent fifteen minutes trying to examine the eyes of an unwashed old bum who kept burping into my face and whose breath smelled as though he had been drinking Lucky Tiger Hair Tonic. Worst of all, I couldn't see a damn thing, which made it difficult for me to do as I had planned, which was to astound the professor by calmly mentioning in an offhand sort of way the previously unnoticed minor finding which would have explained all the poor fellow's medical problems. When the ordeal was over, I crept back to my room and slung the white coat into a corner of the closet. I'd have been much better off wearing a T-shirt and having some knowledge of medical facts and some experience.

At The Vue in the 1960's, the students came, like asparagus, in bunches. Every six weeks a new group arrived on obstetrics and gynecology. They came with eagerness and they came with slothfulness, with innocence and with sophistication, with avarice and with altruism, with amiability and with hostility. Hopefully, they all left knowing at least a little more about the finer and the grosser points of womb-snatching, snatch-patching, and baby-catching. Best of all, several women went home never having even suspected that the young doctors who had carried them through their labors with such solicitous care and then had done such a good job of delivering their babies were medical students. Many a youngster who first saw the light of day at The Vue carries the name of the "doctor" who helped bring him forth. The teachers in the New York schools will never quite figure out Chayim Gonzales or Samuel Rabinowitz Sanchez. But we know, don't we?

As I get older, the different batches of Bellevue students are beginning to blend into each other in my mind's eye. Of course I can still remember that one particular psychotic from 1964 and the impossibly hostile son-of-a-bitch in 1965, and the character who was so incredibly proficient that we suspected him of running an abortion clinic to put himself through school. But I can't distinguish one group from another anymore. Except one. That one I'll remember as long as I live.

Whether fate had simply grouped these guys or whether they had purposely flocked together, I'll never know. But whatever the mechanism, they arrived for their training on the Bellevue obstetrics service during my tenure as a first-year resident.

The obstetrics clinical clerkship for the students at The Vue was the backbreaker of the year. For three weeks, these guys rotated admissions. There were six or seven students in a group, and a student picked up every patient on admission and then followed her to delivery. If she happened to remain in labor for thirty-six hours, no matter. You stayed with your lady until she foaled. Period. This may have accounted for some of the behavior I was privy to during those three weeks, but that's not the whole story. The fact that it only happened in this one group of students makes me a bit suspicious.

Sam Legg was the first one of the group that I met. He was a tall, thin fellow with a perpetually bemused smile and a nervous tic around the mouth. Sam reported for duty, black bag in hand, and I showed him to his patient. I warned him that she was a woman who had already delivered a large number of babies, that she seemed to be in active labor, and that he had therefore better keep a good eye on her. He smiled and said, "Yes, sir!" I told him that he needn't call me sir, that Larry would do fine. He beamed appreciatively, and I ran out to see to the needs of the next customer.

About half an hour later, I heard the kind of screech from the Examining Room that could have meant only one thing. I charged over, pushed through the swinging door, and found myself in total darkness. I groped for the light and, as I switched it on, the woman bellowed again. Sam Legg stood there, opthalmoscope in hand. "Hi, Larry," he smiled. "I had the light off so I could examine her eyes better."

I pushed the patient onto her back so the baby she had been sitting on could get the rest of the way out. Fortunately, no harm had been done. After we completed the delivery, I asked Sam what his findings had been on the pelvic examination. "Gee, Larry," he said. "I never got to the pelvic exam. I was only up to the eyes." For explanation he held up a mimeographed sheet, which I snatched away. It outlined a sample history and physical examination. Sure enough, the pelvic exam was described last.

"Sam," I said. "This is a fine outline. Really it is. But it's not for a medical patient. Since this is obstetrics, you should examine the abdomen and pelvis first."

Apparently there was some mule in Dr. Legg. "This is the sheet they gave us in physical diagnosis," he said. "They told us to stick close to it, and form good habits by practicing that way."

"Sam, let me ask you a question."

"Sure, Larry."

"Suppose you were in the Emergency Room and a guy came in with his jugular vein slashed. Would you check the condition of his eyeballs before you tried to stop the bleeding?"

"No . . . well . . . well, that would be an emergency."

"Couldn't you call this an emergency? A lady delivering a baby sitting on a stretcher while someone is looking at her eyes? And in the dark, yet."

Sam thought for a minute and then allowed that logically it did seem a bit out of order to him. He looked worried. "But how am I going to examine the patients if they deliver first?"

"The fact that they've emptied their uteri doesn't change anything. If they had TB before they delivered, they'll have it afterward too."

A light came on. Sam beamed at me. "Oh—I see. I could do my complete history and physical *after* they deliver." Then he looked worried again. "But wouldn't that be cheating?"

I held onto my composure and assured Sam that it not only would not be cheating, it would be efficient and optimal medical care. So, thereafter, Sam performed his histories and physicals using something resembling the proper priorities. But he often allowed as how it didn't seem quite right to him.

I repeated the story to the chief resident, and expressed some concern for Sam's future functioning as a physician. The chief gently asked me whether I knew that Sam was at that point the top-ranking student in his class. I laughed.

"I'm not kidding," said the chief. "That kid is Numero Uno. So maybe if he tells you something, you ought to listen to him."

I predicted a bright future for Sam Legg as an internist-diagnostician, where he would patiently—and ever so methodically—unravel diagnoses that had stymied lesser minds. I was therefore surprised, to say the least, when a few years ago my wife called my attention to an article written in a popular women's magazine. It was about a set of quintuplets that were born to a woman who had received fertility shots. In describing the woman's delivery, it said, in part, " . . . the first baby was born with the help of the Chief Obstetrical Resident, Dr. Sam Legg . . . " Before me flashed a mental image of a woman sitting in the dark on the edge of a stretcher, surrounded by five writhing babies, while a young doctor peered intently into her eyes.

When I got home after that night's work, I told my wife about my new students. "Thank God it was a slow night," I said. "Only one admission. I wonder what the rest of this group is like."

My wife assured me that I couldn't judge a whole group of students by one member, and that the others probably would be fine. She advised me to cheer up. So I cheered up. I stayed cheerful until I went back to work and met Jack Fields.

Imagine Charlie Brown all grown up and enrolled in medical school. This was Jack Fields. He was short and round-faced, with a light-colored crew cut and a perpetual intimidated little smile. Jack personified the concept of full-fledged wishy-washyness as a religion. For three solid weeks he tortured me. Intravenous solutions didn't get started because Jack stood and wondered whether the vein on the left arm was bigger than the one on the right. Urinalyses were unrecorded because Jack couldn't decide whether the color indicating the quantity of albumen was 1+ or 2+, so he wrote nothing. Women delivered in bed as Jack stood by in paroxysms of inaction. Patients dropped babies off the edges of delivery tables as Jack, standing back where the blood wouldn't drip on him, made feeble passes with his outstretched hands at the emerging infants.

I tried everything I could think of. Pleading, cajoling, cursing, explaining. All gave me the same response: a little-boy smile, and "I'll try harder next time." He did, too. One thing, Jack was not lazy. Incapable, si. Lazy, no.

When Jack's last patient came in, I pulled out my secret weapon: bullying. "Jack," I said, "you work this woman up and take care of her. I will help you not at all. You'd better get the whole works done, and done right." I really hoped that if he were forced to do it—just once—it might be enough.

Fifteen minutes later Jack was back. He held a bloody intravenous catheter in his hand. "I . . . can't start it," he murmured. "Please help me." I waved him back to work. He returned in another ten minutes, holding another bloody catheter. Before he could ask for help, I waved again. Jack stamped his foot and cried out, "I just can't start it. I've used every vein I can see." Then his eyes filled with tears. At that point, I knew we'd both failed.

I took Jack into the resident's room. "Jack," I asked gently. "What the hell are you going to do when you graduate from med school?"

Apparently Jack thought I was offering vocational counseling rather than a commentary with respect to my perception of his inadequacy. "I'm going to be a pediatrician," he said. "I'm going to have my office in the same building where I grew up and still live."

"With your mother and father," I sighed.

Jack brightened. "Yes, that's right," he said. "How did you know?"

God, I was depressed. I could hear the old ladies, who had known him since he was a lad in knickers, burbling at him how nice it would be when he had his own office right there in the apartment building. I saw them patting him on the head. How proud his mother and father must be. How nauseated I was.

Well, a few years ago, our medical school alumni magazine had a squib to the effect that Dr. Jack A. Fields had opened his office for the practice of pediatrics at such-and-such an address in New York. Success was his.

Next to put me to the rack was Herman Morgan. Herman probably was the most enthusiastic person I've ever met. They must have given him the dose of self-confidence and verve that they had withheld from Jack Fields. But as is frequently the case, his outstanding characteristic was both his strong and his weak point.

Herman Morgan could and would do anything. Not only that, he'd invariably do it well. Even better, he was not cursed with that dreadful overconfidence that can lead to one's trying something he really doesn't have the know-how to carry off. In business, that's great; if you fail, you fail. But in medicine, it's the patient who pays the price of such foolhardiness. Herman always knew when to call for help, and it never troubled his ego any to do so.

Now to the debit side: I think that Herman's problem may have only been apparent while he was doing obstetrics. His image is perpetually engraved on my cerebrum, leaning over a woman in labor, up to his armpit in her vagina.

Now I know full well that Herman Morgan really did not do pelvic examinations up to his armpit; that is an anatomic impossibility. But for three weeks I could be anywhere on the labor floor when I'd hear, "Larry! Hey—Larry, com'ere." This would be accompanied by a female shriek of fire-engine proportions. My shoulders would sag and I'd drop what I was doing to go and disimpact Herman from a vagina.

The scene never varied. I'd run into the labor room. Herman would be there, his surgical cap at a jaunty angle, his freckled face bent into an enthusiastic grin, which was accentuated by his widened eyes. His right hand would be lost to view, rammed to the hilt in the birth canal, while the parturient in question was loudly and vigorously trying to wriggle free. The words never varied either, "Hi, Larry. I think she's ready. Would you check me out?"

Herman impressed me as a reasonable man, so I tried to point out to him that his overly vigorous vaginal examinations were both unnecessary and painful. He never failed to be impressed by my descriptions, and would look properly crestfallen. Among his other virtues, Herman was a very kind person, and the last thing he ever intended to do was to hurt a patient. But he got so carried away at the prospect of an imminent delivery that he literally couldn't let go.

After a few of these episodes I gave up. When the call would come resounding through the labor room, I'd just shrug and go to check out Herman. I learned rapidly that he was one of the very few beginning students who were never wrong about an imminent delivery. When he said she was ready, she was indeed ready. So he was a little rough, so what? What the hell, we've all got idiosyncrasies. Maybe it was better that I couldn't cool his enthusiasm. I don't know where Herman Morgan is or what he's practicing, but I am certain he is doing it with vigah.

Immediately after the time I first disengaged Herman Morgan, I staggered out of the room in the direction of the water cooler. On the way I met a new student, a tall, thin serious-looking fellow with horn-rimmed glasses. "All right," I snapped. "What do you do?"

He looked at me with an expression that seemed to say that maybe the dodo wasn't dead after all. "What do you mean?" he asked quietly. "I'm one of the third-year medical students and I just got an admission, so I came to work her up. My name's Louis Schwartz."

"Hello, Louis," I said. "I'm Larry Karp; I'm the resident. What I mean to ask you is what your specialty is."

"I haven't decided yet what I want to go into," he answered.

"That's not what I mean," I said. "In the last night and a half, I have been tortured by a guy who does eye exams in the dark while ladies deliver on the stretchers. I have been set upon by a fellow who has a deathly fear of introducing his fingers into a birth canal, and now I have encountered a grown man who apparently harbors an unsuppressible desire to return to the womb—even one that is already occupied and in which the traffic is moving in the opposite direction. Now I'll ask you again—what is your particular function within this group?"

Louis Schwartz favored me with a smile that was simultaneously knowing and demoniacal. At last he understood.

"I'm the straight man," he said.

The next three weeks proved him to be a man of his word. As the action in the three rings whirled around me, I knew I could always look for Louis. He could be counted on to provide a convenient reference point by which to measure reality. How this one normal individual ended up amid that incredible batch of zanies, I will never know, but I'll be eternally grateful. I don't know what specialty Louis finally chose, but if his year with that gang and his three weeks with me didn't lead him into psychiatry, nothing did.

My encounter with Louis Schwartz reassured me to some extent, but I should have known better. My next recruit was Arturo Gaglione, a very big fellow with shining red cheeks, long wavy hair, and a pair of cheerful, sparkling eyes. Art came into the labor suite and took things over. He did an amazingly efficient job of working up his first patient and got her all set and ready in the labor room in short order. I checked him out and told him to give me a call should he need any help. He cheerfully assured me he would, turned to the patient, and boomed, "This'll get rid of your pain, Mama," zapped her in the arm with a dose of narcotic, and sat himself down at the bedside, his hand on her contracting uterus.

A while later I was finishing up in the delivery room with another student and his patient when a rich baritone voice sang out from the doorway, "Oh, Doc-tor Ka-a-a-rp, oh, Doc-tor Ka-a-a-rp." There was Art standing in the doorway, a grin on his face. I began to wonder where the nearest supply of aspirin was kept. "Yes, Art," I said weakly. "What's up?"

Art threw out his chest and sang again, "Oh, Doc-tor Ka-rp! The baby has come, the baby has come, the baby has come. Lal-la la-la. Yes! Yes!" It sounded rather like a Gilbert and Sullivan production of *La Traviata*. Suddenly even aspirin would have done me no good. I ripped off my delivery gown and went charging past Art into the labor room where his patient had been.

She was lying quietly, cooing into the face of her newborn infant. When she noticed me, she smiled up and said, "You late. D'udda doaktore, he do alla job." Then she smiled at Art Gaglione, who was standing behind me beaming. "He's good doaktore," added the patient. Art just beamed harder.

I restrained my urge to throttle him, primarily because I was certain that as good-natured as he was, under sufficient provocation he'd have been capable of neatly separating me into my component molecules. It turned out, though, that Art really had done a good piece of work. The lady's labor had progressed much faster than he had expected—not an unreasonable thing in view of the fact that this had been his first obstetrical patient—and he suddenly had found himself face to face with the erstwhile fetus. Instead of panicking, fainting, or cutting loose with a screech, any one of which would have been considered *de rigueur* for brand-new students, Art calmly ascertained that I was not going to be of much help to him, so he grabbed hold of our labor room nurse, a former midwife from Jamaica whose delivery skills exceeded those of any resident on the service. Between them they completed the bedside delivery without incident. Only then did Art, flushed with triumph and pride, seek me out.

The reason for his unusual method of announcement, it further developed, was that Art was a raging opera nut. His knowledge of the field was extraordinary, and opera was usually the uppermost thing in his mind. He apparently considered it inappropriate that his moment of glory be celebrated with anything less than a full-fledged aria.

For the rest of the three weeks, I always knew when Arturo Gaglione had a patient in labor. Women labored and babies were born to the accompaniment of choice selections from Mozart, Verdi, Rossini, and Wagner. What the hell, I figured; they say it soothes savage beasts and makes cows give more milk.

The sixth member of the group I have saved for last, not because I met him last, but because all the other lunacies perpetrated by the members of this group paled beside the accomplishments of this one gentleman. Oscar Goldberg could never be encored. There were times when I wondered whether he could even be tolerated.

In retrospect, I think Oscar was simply bored and uninterested in obstetrics. At the time, however, I seriously questioned his sanity. He was a large, lumbering fellow whose shambling walk, thin, unruly hair, and large, protuberant eyes combined to scream DISORGANIZATION at an observer. To say that Oscar was somewhat disorganized would be like saying that Texans are a little boastful. Oscar could never seem to put it all together. One day he'd forget to check a patient's blood pressure. I'd mention this to him, and he'd wholeheartedly agree it was not a good thing to forget. So the next time he'd check the blood pressure, but he'd forget to test the urine. The time after that, it would be the blood count that was missing. Or maybe the birth certificate. One thing I'll say for Oscar, he never made the same mistake twice. But the range of his malfeasances was truly staggering.

His most irritating habit was his wandering. One night I responded to a shriek from a labor room to find a patient lying in the bed, surrounded by blood and amniotic fluid, with her newborn babe doing the Australian crawl between her thighs. After tending to her immediate needs, I went out in search of the culprit. Oscar was pacing slowly down the corridor, eyes up in the air, and hands clasped behind his back. I dragged him into the resident's room for a conference.

He listened quietly to the riot act. "I'm sorry," he said, when I finished. "I just got tired of sitting in there."

I explained that should such be the case, he really ought to arrange for someone to take over temporarily for him. Eyes wide, he promised faithful adherence to the rules in the future.

The next night I looked out into the corridor, and there was Oscar again. I walked over and said hello to him. He glanced at me and said, "Oh, hi. I was just thinking."

"Who's with your patient?" I asked.

"No one," he said. "I just felt like taking a little break."

"Would you like it on the fifth or the sixth rib?" I asked.

He peered at me, totally puzzled. "Huh?"

"Forget it," I said. "Look, Oscar, I thought we agreed that you wouldn't leave your patients alone."

"Well, it shouldn't hurt to take a little break for just a minute."

In our present state of enlightenment, we have learned that to force such issues is fruitless. When faced with latter-day Goldbergs, we try to fill their time on obstetrics with work they will enjoy. A psychiatry-bound student may spend his time interviewing unwed mothers to try to find reasons for contraceptive failures. A budding internist will be assigned to help in the care of those pregnant women with diabetes or heart disease.

However, since in Oscar's day students were still invariably indentured in the labor suite for three weeks, I persevered. At least once nightly I would drag Oscar Goldberg back to his assigned bedside. It became sort of a game. After a while Oscar would see me coming, put his hands behind his head, march back into the labor room, and sit down for a while longer.

Oscar's greatest deed was accomplished one ghastly night when we had in labor a patient with chicken pox pneumonia (who died), a patient with hepatitis (who almost died), and five or eight other women just having babies. About 2 A.M., Oscar's patient foaled. Quickly reviewing the chart, I noticed that she was Rh negative. I drew a tube of blood from her and one from the baby so that the blood bank could test them to see whether she and her baby had incompatible blood types, in which case the baby might have needed a transfusion. I carefully handed the tubes to Oscar. "Take them to the blood bank," I said. "Give them the tech there."

"Sure, Larry," he said.

"And for God's sake, Oscar," I added, "be sure to label which tube is which."

He assured me he would do this, and I went back to see to some of the other patients.

About a half hour later, women were dropping babies right and left, and I was charging back and forth between delivery rooms, when the phone rang. The nurse answered it, and hollered, "Dr. Karp, come and see what this guy wants."

"Jee-sus Christ!" I hollered, and tore over to the desk. Before I had finished saying hello, my eardrum was nearly ruptured by a bellow of "What in holy hell are you doin' up there?"

Now, I was not easily taken aback by odd happenings at Bellevue Hospital, but I will admit that this threw me for a bit of a loss. I thought for an instant and decided to handle the matter with patience and diplomacy. "Who in holy hell are *you*, anyway?" I screamed into the mouthpiece.

It worked. I could hear the gulp at the other end. Then came a forced, controlled voice. "I am the blood bank technician," it said. "And I want to know what is wrong with you crazy bastards up there."

"Why don't you just tell me what's the matter," I said. "I don't know what you're talking about."

"These . . . these . . . these God damn tubes you sent for Rh testing," he spluttered.

The screams of the women and of the students were getting to me. "Christ Almighty, will you tell me what's wrong with them?" I roared. "Aren't they labeled or something?"

"Yes," said the controlled voice. "They're labeled, all right. One is labeled 'Mommy' and the other is labeled, 'Baby.'"

I quietly read the fellow the names and numbers of the patients. Then I went looking for Oscar Goldberg. Fortunately, he had finished up and had gone home to bed. By the time I saw him, the story had already become funny.

After three weeks of this stuff, the students rotated and our new batch arrived. After the first day with the new group, my wife met me at the door. "Do you feel better?" she asked soothingly. "I told you the three weeks would pass."

I slumped into a chair. "Lord," I growled. "What a strait-laced bunch of sourpusses these guys are. They don't do anything funny at all. I thought the day would never pass."

My wife rolled her eyes up in her head and sighed deeply. Then, we sat down to supper.

19

Internship Is Fun and Good for You

The history of medical internship is a saga of privation and suffering.

Until recent years, internship was looked upon as no more than the fifth year of medical education, a time of apprenticeship when the graduate would receive the opportunity to test and refine his new skills under the supervision of experienced physicians. As implied by the name given him, the intern lived in a room on the hospital grounds so that he could be summoned at any hour to meet the needs of his professional charges. Most hospitals, recognizing the basic human requirement for a little R and R, gave each intern one night off duty per week. This largesse did not extend to salaries, though. Since when did people get paid for receiving a valuable education? Only because it was necessary to keep them alive, moving, and relatively odorless, interns were provided free room, board, and laundry services during their year of indenture.

It was primarily the postwar trend toward earlier marriage that altered this general state of affairs. Previously, a married intern had been an unheard-of commodity, but as more and more young medical graduates began to hear the Siren's Song, the age-old foundations began to tremble. Newlyweds established residence in close proximity to the hospitals and let it be known in no uncertain terms that one-night-per-week visits to the love nest were definitely insufficient. Hospital administrators sighed and hired larger numbers of interns, so that an every-other-night work schedule could be established.

That was a start. What came after was truly revolutionary. When those wives found out how their husbands were spending their time, all hell broke loose. "What kind of a game is this?" screeched one intern's mate after another. "Here we live in this cruddy, rat-infested dump, while I work my ass off nursing (or teaching, or sales-clerking), and you don't bring home a plugged nickel."

The interns would blink their bloodshot eyes. "But, dear," they'd answer, "I'm in training."

"Training my ass. What the hell do you think would happen if Bellevue had no interns? Who'd take care of the patients? They'd have to close up."

"Well, I . . . "

"Never mind, 'well I.' Tomorrow you get yourself down to the administrator and tell him you want some money for all that work you do."

In time, the intern staffs got together and paid administration a visit. They suggested it might be nice if they were to receive a wage. The administrators met this idea with a predictable lack of enthusiasm, but the interns reminded them that, after all, they had wives too, and couldn't some little thing be worked out? Eventually the guilt-ridden administrators sat down to work out the details.

By 1963, when I came onto the intern scene, it was pretty well agreed that interns performed a useful and necessary function while they were in the process of obtaining their postgraduate educations. Virtually all hospitals were paying a salary. In some cases, this didn't amount to much. For example, Yale-New Haven doled out $25 a month to their interns. At The Vue, things were considerably better. My salary was $3,200 a year, but an $800 annual "living-out allowance" brought my earnings to a cool $4,000. In combination with Myra's salary as a schoolteacher, this permitted us to rent an apartment where we had a fighting chance against the cockroaches and to eat in such a manner as to avoid coming down with vitamin- and protein-deficiency diseases. Our attending physicians told us how fortunate we were, and how they had *really* had it tough. These comments were guaranteed to earn an older staff man an excessively polite "yes, sir," while more than one junior faculty member was quietly but firmly told to blow it out his ass.

Although judging his training to be first class, no intern at the The Vue could bring himself to feel totally grateful for his lot in life. His day began at about 7:30 A.M., and when it ended at all, it was 6:30 or 7:00 P.M. Sometimes the day did not end: it simply continued through the night until the next evening. Although an occasional blessed ward assignment was associated with an every-third-night rotation, for the greater part of the year the intern was on call every other night. The fact that this worked out to about sixty cents per hour for treating the sickest folks this side of Cook County did little to raise our spirits.

The long hours did even less for our educations than for our morale. One psychologist after another has determined that after someone has been awake for twenty-four consecutive hours, he's only slightly more capable of learning something than he is of taking off from the roof of The Vue and soaring gracefully over the canyons of lower Manhattan. Sleeplessness thoroughly wipes out the ability to concentrate and greatly impairs the power of recall. In addition, by about the thirtieth hour out of the sack, you generally find yourself not particularly caring whether anyone lives or dies—including, and sometimes especially, yourself.

So it was that I came down to mid-February of my internship year in a sorry condition. It had been a hard winter in New York, with much cold weather and appreciable quantities of the white stuff that causes poets to burst forth with paeans. The Bowery citizens were being admitted in flocks. For the past four months, the only thing around The Vue that had been fuller than the wards were my nights. Under the best of circumstances, it was not customary to be able to snatch more than two or three hours of sleep during a night on call, but at that point it seemed like it had been weeks since my on-call bed and I had renewed our acquaintance. It seemed like weeks because it had been weeks.

An insidious thing began to happen to me. After their nights off, interns do not exactly leap from their beds, pound their chests, and do twenty deep-knee bends. But they do manage to get up, feeling more or less ready for the upcoming thirty-six big ones. Only in retrospect did I realize that I was losing my resilience. Where I formerly had managed to get out of bed five minutes after the alarm went off, it became ten minutes, and then fifteen. It stayed at fifteen minutes only because, at that point, my wife would apply her icy feet to my back and push. Then I'd stagger into the bathroom, feeling as though I would throw up any minute, and when I'd look in the mirror to shave, I'd have to operate among and between a field of little black dancing dots.

By the time I came home from work, I'd be utterly wiped out.

I'd go into the bedroom to change out of my white uniform before supper, and more often than not, my wife would come in a few minutes later to find me lying on the bed on my back, my bare legs hanging over the edge. This happened because I'd sit on the bed to take off my pants and simply fall over backward, sound asleep. One evening she discovered me with my right leg up in the air, flexed at both the knee and the ankle, my hands arrested in the process of taking off the sock. Why I was doing that, we haven't figured out to this day.

Once aroused and having eaten supper, I suffered through bouts of the greatest ambivalence I've ever experienced. I had to decide whether I should go directly to bed and recoup as much of my loss as possible. Or should I keep myself awake, by self-torture if necessary, just to enjoy the unalloyed pleasure of knowing I was off duty? Worst of all were the free weekend days. I could easily have slept till four in the afternoon on every one of them, but it seemed absolutely criminal not to be awake and ecstatic every possible moment I wasn't at The Vue. So I'd set the alarm for around noon, thereby splitting the difference, and causing me to feel generally dissatisfied with myself.

Other peculiar things occurred. I'd leave the apartment to go to work and suddenly find myself inside The Vue without being able to recall the process of having gotten there. I didn't think much of it at the time. We all have episodes of that sort of automatic behavior, and they're perfectly normal. While driving a car along a freeway, we may suddenly realize that we're ten miles nearer our destination, but can't recall any of the intervening scenery. We've been concentrating on some thought or another to the exclusion of all else, using subconscious mechanisms to steer the car. But again, in retrospect, I realize that I never had the foggiest notion as to what concepts had been temporarily possessing my mind with such ferocity as to shut out all the magnificent sights between Stuyvesant Town and The Vue.

I began to forget other things as well, and got into the habit, which I haven't shaken to this day, of writing myself notes and lists. Less acute problems went into my shirt pocket, while must-do-nows were clipped to my tie bar. Only in this way could I remember that it was Mrs. Gonzalez who needed the penicillin and Mrs. Goldberg who required the enema, and not the other way around.

Lincoln's Birthday was a holiday at The Vue and, to celebrate, we went to lunch at the Philippine Gardens. This was a little place a few blocks away where, for under three dollars two could stuff themselves to bursting with first-class Filipino cooking. I say we went there that day because Myra tells me we did. I have no recollection of the event. The meal was made memorable for my wife, she says, by my incessant yawning. She finally grew weary of studying my tonsilar beds and requested that I cover my mouth. Whereupon, eager to please, I suppose, I put my hand over my eyes, leaving my mouth unabashedly agape. My wife and the other couple we were with enjoyed a merry laugh over my little bit of silly behavior. At least I'm told they did.

At about this time, I came to the decision that sleep was more important than food, and so, every day when the other interns went down for lunch, I would forgo Miz Matthews' delicacy of the day and hightail it for my room. There, I'd carefully set the clock radio for half an hour in the future, turn up the volume full blast, and proceed to savor thirty indescribably delicious minutes of sleep. The alarm always seemed to go off almost as soon as I had set it, and I'd drag myself to my feet by sheer power of will, drop past the cafeteria and belt down a couple of slices of bread or a candy bar, and head up to the ward for the afternoon's work.

The whole thing came to a head on a dismal Friday afternoon. The temperature was right around freezing and the remains of a recent New York snowfall lay on the curbs, gray and disgusting. I had had no sleep the night before and relief was still not in sight. Remember, we worked essentially every other night. The word "essentially" is important: in order to be able to get a full weekend off duty, we'd work Thursday, Thursday night, Friday, and Friday night. Then, at noon Saturday, we'd be gloriously free till Monday morning, while the other intern covered the ward. So another full twenty-four hours of sleeplessness lay before me. I was not pleased.

During rounds that morning, I had been unusually irritable. I peevishly questioned the necessity of every therapeutic maneuver suggested by Ellen Carlyle, our resident. The last bed we stopped at belonged at the time to Mrs. Greenspan, an eighty-some-year-old woman who had been brought to The Vue two weeks before, unconscious from a stroke. Unresponsive she had come, and unresponsive she remained, a most ominous prognosis. Ellen solicited suggestions regarding her care. I recommended that we notify her family not to let her insurance policy lapse and then arrange to let her incubate her bedsores in a nursing home. Ellen told me, a bit tartly, that she didn't think I was very funny. I didn't care.

I spent the rest of the morning working on the ward and, when lunchtime came, I made my customary scoot upstairs to my room, set the alarm, and let my eyelids snap shut. Just another twenty-four hours . . .

I still don't remember the alarm going off, and I have no recollection whatever of getting out of the bed. Neither is there a memory of walking down to the ward, but somehow or other I got there. I was sitting at the desk, with the patients' order book open in front of me and my pen in my hand, when I was seized by overwhelming uncertainty. Several times I started to write my order, but I knew there was something peculiar about it. Then I began to feel generally confused, a very unpleasant sensation.

I looked around and saw Ellen standing across the room, in front of the doorway to the examining cubicle. Slowly I got up, carrying the order book, and walked over to her.

"Are you sure you want me to give that dextroamphetamine to Mrs. Greenspan?" I asked.

Now I was not the only confused person in the room. She put one hand on her hip and stared up at me. "Larry, what in the world are you talking about?" she said, with just the least bit of edginess in her voice.

Suddenly I felt completely exasperated. Here I was, working like hell, and people were playing games with me. "Come on," I growled. "Quit crapping around. Not five minutes ago on rounds, you told me to give Greenspan a slug of Dex. But I just don't think it's a very good idea."

Ellen looked even more confused. She held out her wrist. "We finished rounds at a quarter after ten this morning," she said, very evenly.

I looked first at her watch and then at my own. They both said one-thirty.

My heart started to pound and my cheeks began to burn. "B— but . . . you . . . I know you said . . . At that point, confusion totally overwhelmed me and words failed. I had an urge to run from the room.

My expression must have revealed my emotions, because Ellen took me by the arm and led me back across the room to the desk. "Sit down here a minute, Larry," she said. "Just wait here for me.

I'll be right back, and we'll straighten this all out." She stared hard into my eyes.

I nodded.

"Promise you won't get up till I come back."

"I'll wait," I said. I no longer wanted to run. The panic was still there, but it had become paralyzing. I felt afraid to do or say anything.

Ellen flew out of the ward and came back, almost immediately, it seemed, with the chief resident. "Tell Bob what's bothering you," she said.

I hesitated, and then, suddenly, the words came out in a stream. "Well, on rounds Ellen told me to give Mrs. Greenspan a dose of Dexedrine to wake her up but the more I think about it the sillier it sounds because Dexedrine won't wake up an old lady out of a stroke and for all I know it might even kill her but somehow it got to be one-thirty right after rounds were over and I don't understand it."

Bob and Ellen looked at each other, and I got even more scared. "What the hell is going on?" I asked, not at all certain I wanted an answer.

"I'm not sure," Bob said, very gently. "Let's go down the hall and talk to Dr. Kalb."

Dr. Kalb was the associate chairman of the department of medicine, and was in charge of the training program. If I had been frightened before, I was terrified now.

"Don't worry," Bob said. "No sweat. We'll have this all straightened out in no time. Come on, let's go."

Dr. Kalb listened patiently to the three-part recitative, tapping the eraser end of a pencil against his desk and smiling faintly in the manner of a man who knows exactly what's coming. I envied him intensely. When we had finished talking, he leaned back in his chair and folded his hands across his belly. "Tell me something," he said, looking at me. "Have you been up a lot at night during the past few weeks?"

I started to laugh. I knew it wasn't appropriate, but I couldn't help it. I fought to get myself under control, and finally managed to choke out the information that I hadn't seen my bed during the last three weeks of call.

Dr. Kalb nodded. Suddenly he barked out, "What did you have for lunch today?"

I began to stammer, and as I did, the true state of affairs

popped into my head. I quickly explained my recently acquired habit of midday nap-taking. "So I must have dreamed that Ellen told me to give that old lady the Dexedrine," I said. But then, the doubts regrouped. "Problem is," I muttered, "it still seems real to me, not a dream. And I still don't remember getting up and going down to the ward."

"You're suffering from the sleep-deprivation syndrome," Dr. Kalb said. "Go on home and go right to bed. You'll be as good as ever in a couple of days."

I was horrified. Go home? If I were to do that, another intern would have to cover for me. The ultimate crime! Two years before, an intern had nearly died because he had insisted upon carrying out his duties in spite of a severe stomachache. The next day they took him directly from his ward to the operating room and removed his burst appendix.

"I'll be okay now," I said quickly. "I'll just stay awake until tomorrow morning, so I won't be able to have any more dreams; then I'll go to bed for the weekend." It seemed very logical to me.

Dr. Kalb tried as delicately as he could to lead me to understand that my judgment was sufficiently impaired that I could not be trusted with the care of patients. However, he was in a situation right out of *Catch-22*. My judgment was indeed in a bad way, and as a result, I didn't believe him. Had I been of sound judgment, of course, I'd have understood at once. But then, there would have been no need for him to be talking to me in the first place.

In any event, Dr. Kalb really went out of his way not to upset me. He could have told me to simply get my ass out of his office and into my bed, that I was summarily relieved of duties till further notice. But instead he asked, almost casually, "You believe that Dr. Cohen knows his business, don't you?"

My judgment was not so far gone that I could say no. Dr. Henry Cohen had been trained in both neurology and psychiatry, and was universally acclaimed at The Vue as the most competent and rational of all possible Shrinks. I said yes.

"Good," said Dr. Kalb. "I'm going to call him now. Then, you go and talk to him. If he says you can work, then it's fine with me. But if he says you should go home, then you'll go. Fair enough?"

I nodded smugly. How could Dr. Cohen say I was unfit to work just because I was a little tired?

"Dr. Kalb is as right as he can be," said Dr. Cohen, after he had listened to me tell my story for the fourth time. "You absolutely have got to get some sleep, and right away."

I was crushed. Before I knew what was happening, tears started to run down my cheeks.

"What's wrong?" asked Dr. Cohen. "Why should an intern cry when someone tells him to go to bed?"

I wiped at my eyes, but to my annoyance and embarrassment, the waterworks flowed on. I explained how sad it was making me to think that because of my dereliction, another intern was going to have to do double work.

For a few minutes Dr. Cohen remained quiet. He seemed to be thinking. "Try to understand," he finally said. "Look how unstable your emotions are. You know that's not normal. But it fits right in with the sleep-deprivation syndrome. You know, people are funny. If you happened to have caught pneumonia, and were running a temperature of 103°, you'd get right into bed and stay there until you were better. Well, let me tell you: you're no less sick at this moment than a patient with pneumonia, and you're no less in need of treatment. If it makes you feel any better, you're not in the least unique. Once a year we go through this business. That's right: every year, one intern manages to get so little sleep that he collapses. Or has delusions. Or hallucinates. And do you think we can ever manage to convince him what's wrong? Every time, Kalb has to call me up to act as the arbiter. So don't feel guilty. There's nothing fundamentally wrong with you. You just happen to have pulled the short straw for this year."

I took a deep breath. "What do you want me to do?" I asked.

"Get all the sleep you can between now and Monday morning," said Dr. Cohen. "Then come back and see me."

"Then can I go back to work?"

"Then we'll talk about it. Go home."

Myra was a little alarmed when she came home from work and found me curled up like a fetus on one of the living room chairs. She was not reassured when I gave her the fifth recitation of my lengthening story of sleeplessness.

"Why aren't you asleep, then?" asked my wife.

"I'm too hungry to sleep," I said. Actually, I hadn't wanted her to come home and find me inexplicably sacked out. I don't know why I didn't just say that.

"So why didn't you get something to eat?"

"I never thought of it," I said lamely.

Myra looked at me in a peculiar tone of voice. "I'll get you a sandwich," she said. She did, and I ate it ravenously. I realized I actually was very hungry. Then, I went to bed. It was 4:30 in the afternoon.

When I opened my eyes, the room was still light. At least I thought it was still light. But when I looked at the clock radio and saw that it was 2:30, I realized that it actually was *again* light, and I had slept for twenty-two hours. Furthermore, I'm quite certain that the only reason I woke up even then was because my bladder was threatening to rupture. Bent over double, I made my way to the bathroom and urinated for what seemed like five minutes.

Myra appeared at the door in midstream. "You're alive," she said.

"Very funny." My head was both pounding and swimming, and I was not amused.

"No kidding," she insisted. "A couple of times I went in to feel your pulse. You didn't move for hours at a stretch, and there were times when I wasn't sure you were breathing."

I ate some cereal and toast, and then we sat and talked for a while. Before long, I began to yawn uncontrollably, and this symptom, together with the headache and dizziness, impressed upon me the undeniable fact that I ought to go back to sleep. So I did. This time I slept only till noon on Sunday, a stretch of a mere nineteen hours. Out of a total of forty-four consecutive hours, I had been awake three. I managed to remain conscious until nine Sunday evening, and then conked out again until the alarm roused me at eight Monday morning.

By nine I was in Dr. Cohen's office. He asked me how I felt, and I could truthfully tell him much better, even though I hadn't felt bad the past Friday. As I looked back, though, I realized how foggy and confused I had been. I asked whether I might return to work.

Dr. Cohen held up his hand. "Let's do an EEG first," he said.

The electroencephalogram was a scary thing. They stuck little needles under my scalp; the needles were attached to wires which led to a recording apparatus which, in turn, traced out the patterns of the electrical activity in different parts of my brain. I couldn't help conjuring up an image of myself, with wires coming out of a machine and disappearing into my scalp. I knew that the flow of information was from me to the machine, but how could I be sure they weren't going to reverse polarities and give me electroshock, or maybe even reprogram my cerebrum?

"That's typical of the sleep-deprivation syndrome, too," said Dr. Cohen, when I told him my reaction to the EEG. He smiled. "That's really a pretty paranoid thought, when you come right down to it. Prolonged sleeplessness often brings on some very impressive reactions."

Disappointment began to build up in my throat. "You mean I'm not better yet?"

"No, I do think you're better," said Dr. Cohen. "But you're certainly not ready to go back to work. Look. You slept twenty-two hours, nineteen hours, and eleven hours, and the only reason you stopped at eleven was that you set an alarm so you'd be able to come and see me." He held up the EEG tracing, a long, thin line of what to me were indecipherable jumps and squiggles. "Your tracing still shows some of the changes we see with sleep deprivation--but they're non-specific sorts of things. There's certainly nothing to worry about: no sign of organic disease, no tumor or anything like that. Just go on back home and sleep until you can't sleep anymore. Come see me again Friday."

"Friday?" I screeched.

"Friday," Dr. Cohen calmly echoed. "It'll take that long to get you back into condition."

"That's ridiculous," I snapped, without thinking.

Dr. Cohen smiled wanly. "Dr. Karp," he said laconically. "Let me appeal to the sense of logic you've undoubtedly regained since last week. Since when has Bellevue Hospital ever in any way coddled an intern?"

I turned around and went home. By the time Myra returned from work, I had already put in six and a half blissful hours and was still going strong.

That night I slept only fourteen hours, and twelve each of the next two. The feeling of drawing achiness vanished from my thighs and calves, and the inside of my head felt almost painfully clear. Thursday night, I needed just nine and a half hours, and Friday morning Dr. Cohen gave me the go-ahead to come back to work the following Monday. I did, and managed to finish out the remainder of my internship year without trouble.

In 1956, eight years before I fell victim to the sleep-deprivation syndrome, Dr. Salvatore Cutolo, the deputy administrator of The Vue wrote:

> In all my years at Bellevue I've never heard a doctor complain about being overworked. Quite the opposite, in fact. I hear grumbling when the hospital census drops and there isn't *enough* to stimulate the imagination of our interns. They never consider their work here in the light of earning a livelihood. They are rounding and completing their educations.

It's utterly incomprehensible to me how Dr. Cutolo could never have heard an intern complain about being overworked. We bitched about it endlessly. We bitched on the wards; we bitched in the halls. We bitched in the dining room, in the elevators, and in the bathrooms. One of my roommates even bitched in his sleep. We bitched about it to anyone who would give half an ear. But then, Dr. Cohen had put it very well: The Vue was never known to coddle an intern in any imaginable way.

However, the question still remains: *Should* interns work those hours? It used to be that whenever the issue arose, the elders would shut off discussion with a simple, "It's the only way to learn medicine. We survived, and you'll survive, too."

Well, it may not be the only way to learn medicine; in fact, it may not even be the best. And the interns may survive, but the patients may not. A couple of years ago, an article in the *New England Journal of Medicine* reported that after a full day and night on call, interns could be shown to be suffering from serious defects in both judgment and cognitive abilities. Studies of this sort can't be ignored forever, and therefore I think it's likely that eventually doctors-in-training will find themselves working on a shift basis, which will provide them the opportunity to get necessary amounts of sleep on a regular basis. It won't be like the good old days, but maybe that's not the most important consideration.

20

Everything's Up-to-Date at The Vue

The members of the Bellevue house staff employed only the most modern of medical practices. Nothing but current theories and principles were utilized. The local version of the game of one-up consisted of trying to outdo your competitors in quoting facts and figures from recent issues of medical journals.

Like all young people, we suffered from a disease called Severe History Deficiency. We shuddered at the barbaric practices of our ancestors, but naturally we never gave much thought to the mental discomfort we would ourselves one day cause our descendants.

A mere hundred years before my time at The Vue, the famous British obstetrician John Braxton Hicks introduced a new, less-traumatic method for turning a fetus around inside the uterus. By the use of his technique, he was able to reduce the maternal mortality associated with placenta previa (a placenta implanted very low in the uterus, so as to block the birth canal) from 30 to 5 percent, surely a remarkable achievement. Hicks became justly famous in his day.

In that day, caesarean section was probably the deadliest of all surgical operations. Every caesarean section performed in Paris between 1787 and 1876 resulted in the death of the mother. It was safer to be delivered via the goring of a bull than by the surgeon's knife. In New York City in 1887, angry bulls tore open the uteri of nine women; five of the victims survived. Yet only one of the eleven women subjected to caesarean section in that year in that city lived to labor another day. Small wonder that the caesarean operation came to be used only as a desperate last resort, frequently when the patient was moribund.

207

However, time passed, and as it did, modern obstetrical practice changed. Obstetricians learned how to properly suture a uterine incision, and then they picked up a few timely hints on cleanliness from Dr. Pasteur and Dr. Lister. Suddenly caesarean section gained not only respectability but respect. Therapeutic horizons undreamed of in the ancient days of Braxton Hicks opened up to the most mediocre of early twentieth-century obstetricians.

Now, when a placenta was thoughtless enough to implant low in the uterus, blocking the baby's path of descent, one had only to cut into the organ from above, extract the child alive, and set matters generally aright. Not only did this mode of therapy have the advantage of expedition, but it also permitted the operator to avoid the risks of uterine rupture or exsanguinating hemorrhage which attended the vaginal manipulations (including Braxton Hicks's version) formerly necessary in the management of placenta previa. The maternal mortality associated with this complication plunged to one percent, and after blood transfusion became established as a routine procedure, mortality fell even further, approaching one case in 1,000. By the time I began my residency, there wasn't a modern obstetrician alive who would have been caught dead doing a Braxton Hicks version. The watchword of the faith had become "When in doubt, cut it out."

Thus the modern obstetrician of 1964 resorted to caesarean section far more readily than did his predecessor. But old customs die hard. There was still a tendency to look upon a section as representing a failure in a sense: a slightly shameful inability to deliver the baby from below. This attitude originated in the days when caesarean section was just beginning to come to the fore. Older obstetricians were proud of their hard-acquired ability to perform all sores of intrauterine gymnastics.

Thus the advent of caesarean section was gradual, the frequency of use increasing as more young graduates went out into practice, replacing the old-timers being transferred to the Great Labor Room in the Sky. But the criticisms of their professional fathers remained in the ears of the new doctors, causing them to wonder just a bit over the propriety of every section they did. This vague inborn guilt was transmitted to the next generation of obstetricians, and to the one after that. So, even in the early 1960's the excellence of an obstetrics service was still being judged in part by the number of caesarean sections it had been found necessary to perform. Any figure over 3 percent caused eyebrows to shoot skyward and suggestions to be made that perhaps the doctors were getting a little knife-happy. This lingering suspicion surrounding caesarean section was responsible for some pregnancy outcomes which at the time seemed unfortunate but unavoidable. In retrospect though, they make me squirm much as I suspect Braxton Hicks must have wriggled in his chair in 1861 when he thought about the techniques he had previously used to turn fetuses.

For example, there was the case of Eufemia Montalvo. Mrs. Montalvo was a jolly, smiling Puerto Rican who packed two hundred pounds onto her five-two frame. She came to The Vue in labor one heady spring evening when the perfume from the East River garbage scows was wafting through the open windows of the labor and delivery suite. She told me her pains had begun a few hours earlier, her waters had not yet broken, and volunteered the opinion that this labor seemed just like her previous two. But it wasn't. A glance at her prenatal-care record told me that her two children had been born, as are most children head-first. This fetus, however, was coming either ass-backward or ass-forward, depending upon how you define your terms. It was presenting by the breech.

In 1965, at The Vue, when a mother was unable to push out a breech baby by dint of her own efforts, the child was usually extracted. This procedure involved reaching up, grabbing the baby's feet, and then pulling it into the world. The chance to do a breech extraction was an opportunity highly prized by senior residents, so I called Bryan Rollins, my second-year man. He, in turn, called Guillermo Sueza, the third-year resident. Together we reviewed Mrs. Montalvo's situation.

We all agreed that she had a breech presentation. We differed a little, though, on our estimates of the baby's weight. Under the best of circumstances, this is difficult to appraise accurately, and Mrs. Montalvo's more-than-adequate padding made the circumstances anything but the best. Guillermo and I both estimated the weight at around eight and a half pounds, but Bryan said he thought it was more like nine and a half. He shook his head. "Gonna be a tight squeeze," he said.

Guillermo laughed and shook his head. "Won't be any problem," he said. "You just do a good breech extraction, it comes right out. I'll help you. You do it, and I'll help you with it."

Bryan looked dubious. "It's a mighty big baby," he said.

Guillermo picked up the prenatal record. "Look," he said. "Her first baby weighed nine-two, and her second one was nine-five. She delivered both of them without any kind of trouble. Her pelvis must be plenty big."

Bryan looked only slightly reassured. He scratched his head and mumbled, "Yeah, I guess you're right."

"Sure," said Guillermo, and slipped me a wink. "You just got to do the extraction right, that's all. You're always worrying too much."

Bryan bit his lower lip. "Okay," he said, and turned to me. "Call us when she's ready to deliver."

"You bet," I said.

Over the next two hours, I gave Mrs. Montalvo the hawk-eye treatment. I knew that if I failed to watch her closely, and didn't give Bryan and Guillermo sufficient time to get down to the floor, scrub up, and get gowned, they would be more than a little angry with me. And justifiably so.

When at last the two senior residents marched into the delivery room, all ready to extract, I had the patient up in stirrups, with the anesthetist sitting by her head. Both senior residents examined the patient and agreed that her cervix was completely dilated. All that remained was for the baby to be pushed and/or pulled through the birth canal.

I felt the uterus begin to tighten under my hand. "She's having a contraction," I called out.

"Push, Mama," said Bryan, leaning forward from the bottom of the delivery table. "Push as hard as you can. Push, push, push, push, push, push, push, push!"

Mrs. Montalvo strained against the handles on the sides of the table. Her face turned bright red and the veins on her neck stood out like blue worms. Her anus bulged, releasing a large piece of stool which plopped into the bucket at the foot of the table. Finally, her contraction over, her head fell back onto the table, and she panted and gasped for breath.

"Good push," said Bryan to Guillermo. "But she didn't move the baby a bit."

"Okay," said Guillermo. "Let's do the extraction, then." He asked the anesthetist to put her to sleep.

While the anesthesia was being administered, Bryan and Guillermo carefully reviewed the technique of breech extraction;

during the procedure, there would be no opportunity to rectify a false move. Then, as soon as the patient had been rendered unconscious, Bryan cautiously inserted his hand into the vagina. "Got both feet," he muttered. As he pulled downward, the feet appeared at the vulva. They looked big.

Bryan kept pulling, and the baby's rump came out, followed by the back. A couple of twists and the shoulders were free. Then, Guillermo took hold of the feet as Bryan made ready to deliver the head. The umbilical cord hung down in a loop from the middle of the abdomen.

Bryan put one hand over the nape of the baby's neck, slipped a finger of the other into the mouth, and began to pull. I leaned over Mrs. Montalvo's abdomen to watch the head emerge, but nothing happened. Well, not exactly nothing. Bryan's face turned bright red, and drips of sweat fell from his forehead onto the baby's back.

"It won't come," he said, looking back at Guillermo.

"Wiggle it a little," said Guillermo.

Bryan wiggled, but the head still didn't budge. Guillermo felt the umbilical cord to count the heart rate. "It's down to sixty," he said. "Better put on the Pipers."

I ran across the room and came back with a pair of Piper forceps, an instrument specially designed for the extraction of the aftercoming head of a breech baby. His hands shaking more than a little, Bryan took the forceps, applied them, and pulled downward, at first gingerly, and then with all his might.

"Jesus Christ," he moaned. "The God-damn thing's absolutely stuck tight."

"The cord's not beating now," said Guillermo rapidly. "We gotta get the baby out fast. Here, gimme the Pipers."

He exchanged places with Bryan, took a deep breath, braced his feet against the table, and yanked. I felt sick to my stomach as I heard the unmistakable crunch of breaking bone. With that, the head of the baby flew out of the vagina, sending Guillermo staggering backward a couple of steps. Recovering himself, he began to slap the limp baby's feet.

"Forget it," said Bryan dully, rubbing his hand lightly over the crushed, flattened back of the baby's head.

Guillermo turned pale above his mask as he looked up and saw what Bryan was showing him. Without another word, he clamped and cut the umbilical cord, and placed the baby into the bassinet. When we weighed it later, the scale read ten pounds, six ounces.

Our management of this case constituted good, standard obstetrical practice in 1965, but obstetricians have now come to realize that when large babies present by the breech, it's much safer to deliver them by caesarean section. In the case of a head presentation, several hours may safely elapse while the head gradually works its way through the mother's pelvis, but the aftercoming head of a breech baby must descend through the pelvis in just a couple of minutes. And with the rest of the child already born, there can be no turning back when the head hangs up, as occurred in the unfortunate case of Mrs. Montalvo.

As with the Braxton Hicks version, a breech extraction can be a real ego trip for the obstetrician, much more so than a caesarean section. But only when the extraction is successful. Guillermo and Bryan didn't feel any too good for several days after Mrs. Montalvo's delivery. As judged by contemporary standards, their actions had given them no reason to feel guilty, but doctors customarily look upon the death of a patient as representing failure, and take the matter very much to heart.

In some respects, Marta Garcia's case resembled Mrs. Montalvo's. It would have taken two Martas to make one Eufemia, though. Mrs. Garcia was a slightly-built-nineteen-year-old Puerto Rican who came to The Vue in labor with her first child. As the labor progressed, it became obvious that she had the Puerto Rican problem: a flat pelvis.

Since the Puerto Ricans who emigrated from their sunny isle to the Lower East Side of New York were overwhelmingly from the poorest segment of Caribbean society, their nutrition had been none too good while they were growing up. Consequently, they suffered from a generalized softening of their bones. One consequence of this condition was that the developing pelvic bones became excessively molded so that the pelvis was extremely flattened from front to back. Then, in labor, the short pelvic dimensions would block the passage of the baby.

Thus, Mrs. Garcia labored bravely, but in futility. Her cervix dilated properly, but the baby couldn't descend through the birth canal. I called the senior resident for the night, Peter Edwards. Pete came down, examined Mrs. Garcia, and rubbed his hands together in eager anticipation. It was a case for the Bartons.

The Barton forceps was an instrument designed to fit into a flat pelvis and extract the baby. Because of the large number of these architecturally deformed birth canals that found their way into The Vue, the Bartons had achieved great popularity there, and the residents were all eager to use it. Like a successful breech extraction, a good Barton delivery was a real ego trip.

When it became apparent that Mrs. Garcia had pushed her baby as far down as she possibly could, we took her to the delivery room, gave her a spinal anesthetic, and put her up in the stirrups for delivery. Pete put on his gown and gloves, did a careful last-minute examination, and applied the Bartons. Then he got down on one knee and began to pull.

I say he pulled. He tugged. He yanked. He towed. He hauled and wrenched. His efforts made Bryan's attempt with the Pipers seem feeble by comparison. Great torrents of sweat flooded his eyes and his ears and formed lakes on the floor in front of him. What we could see of his face was the color of an overripe tomato, and the veins on his neck bulged frighteningly.

After what seemed like half an hour, but was really more like five minutes, the baby emerged. No one in the room was breathing including the baby. After Barton extractions, not many newborns demonstrated terribly much in the way of spontaneous respiration.

We all set to work resuscitating the infant, while Pete sewed up Mrs. Garcia so that she once again looked as her Creator had intended. After about five minutes of oxygen and other indicated tonics, the baby started to come around. By fifteen minutes, he was breathing on his own, and by half an hour, he was obviously no longer in danger.

So Mrs. Garcia got to take home a live baby. However, by today's standards, we really may not have done her a favor. We've learned that babies who are severely depressed at birth often don't do as well as expected on IQ tests and neurological examinations later in life. For this reason, difficult forceps extractions, which may cause neonatal depression, have been largely supplanted by caesarean sections which, although less exciting, seem to yield up babies in much better condition.

In 1965, the standard technique for evaluating the well-being of a baby during labor was to listen periodically to its heartbeat through the mother's abdomen, using an especially sensitive stethoscope. This approach, identical to the procedures of a hundred years earlier, was really less than satisfactory. Listening times were short, usually a minute or less, and during the non-auscultatory intervals of five to fifteen minutes, much damage could and sometimes did occur.

The relative insufficiency of the fetuscope was illustrated by my experience with Lucy Romero and her fetus. Like Marta Garcia, Lucy was nineteen and in labor for the first time. But she was an unusual Bellevue patient in a few respects. First, she spoke flawless English. Second, she was unusually poised and mature. And third, she had a husband with her. This was most unusual of all.

A large number of the obstetrical patients at The Vue had no husbands, period. But even those who were married came to labor alone. Sometimes the husband stayed home with the kids; other times, he was reported to be out drinking with his friends. We were told by the Puerto Rican hospital personnel that it simply was not the custom in the Commonwealth for husbands to wait out labor at the hospital: it was considered weakly sentimental and even a bit unseemly.

In a year as resident in obstetrics and gynecology, I encountered exactly one husband who sat through his wife's labor, and that was Pedro Romero. He was all of twenty, but like his wife, mature and well spoken. The reason for his exceptional behavior soon became clear: both Pedro and Lucy were not native Puerto Ricans. They had been born and raised on the Lower East Side. Thus they had had full opportunity to absorb all sorts of American customs.

This was before Lamaze had become a household word, though, and Pedro did not actually sit *with* Lucy during her labor. Except for brief visits, husbands and other relatives were not permitted on the labor floor. So Pedro paced the corridor outside labor and delivery while Lucy labored within.

Since she was not far along when she arrived, I told Pedro to put on a gown and come in. I figured it was going to be a long wait. He tiptoed into the labor room, pulled up a chair at Lucy's bedside, and took her hand. As she had her next contraction, she squeezed his hand and moaned softly. All the color drained out of poor Pedro's cheeks. As soon as the pain had passed, he stood up. "I think I *will* wait outside, Doctor, if you don't mind," he said. "I don't like to see her having pain."

After I had ushered him to the corridor, I went back and sat down next to Lucy. It was a slow night. She was my only patient, and for the first time I was feeling like a private obstetrician. I coached her through her contractions and gave her medication when she needed it. Periodically, I checked her progress, and then afterwards, excused myself and went outside to give a report to Pedro. His response was invariable: a smile and "Thank you, Doctor. Sounds like it's going pretty good."

As a matter of fact, it *was* going pretty good. Lucy made rapid progress in dilating the cervix, and by six hours after her admission, she was ready to try to push the baby down and out. With each contraction, I encouraged her to push, which she did very well. Between contractions, as she lay back in bed to rest, I listened to the heartbeat of the fetus. It was perfectly regular, and at just the right rate.

A half hour of pushing went by, and the baby was descending right on schedule; I figured that with another fifteen or thirty minutes of work, she'd be ready for an easy delivery. As her latest contraction wore off, I picked up the fetuscope, placed the end of the instrument on her abdomen, and listened.

I couldn't hear the fetal heartbeat.

My first reaction was confusion; I checked to make certain I was listening in the right place. That issue was easily resolved, because I had marked an X on the belly at the spot where the heart sounds could be heard most easily. Then I moved the scope around, but I still couldn't hear anything. Even allowing for the possibility that the baby had moved significantly lower in the birth canal didn't help.

Meanwhile, another contraction had begun. Lucy pushed with all her might. When the contraction passed, I listened again. All I got was the same deafening silence.

Now my mind was made up. I knew that babies born without heartbeats can sometimes be revived, and I also knew that Lucy's baby was low enough in the pelvis that it could be safely delivered with forceps. Quickly I explained the situation to Lucy as I simultaneously began to move her toward the delivery room. I thought about giving a report to Pedro, but decided against the idea, mostly because I didn't want to take the time.

The nurse put Lucy up for delivery, and as rapidly as I could, I applied the forceps to the baby's head. Then I cut an episiotomy sufficient to permit passage of one of Mr. Mack's largest. The baby practically fell out into my hands. My heart was playing a drum roll.

As it turned out, so was the baby's heart. The kid came out howling; it couldn't have been in better condition. I put it into the bassinet and then spent the next forty-five minutes sewing Lucy's bottom back together.

Why hadn't I heard the heartbeat? I still can't be sure. It's possible, but very unlikely, that the heart really had stopped and that the shock of the forceps application and pull started it up again. It's much more probable that the baby actually had moved within the uterus so as to shift the point of transmission of the heartbeat, and I simply had failed to place the fetuscope in the proper place.

It was weeks before Lucy could sit without a foam cushion under her, but she didn't care, because she figured it had been necessary to save her baby. As much as I tried to explain that I had probably just been mistaken, she didn't listen.

Neither did Pedro. Lucy told her husband of my wondrous deed, and the next evening, he came looking for me. He brushed aside my explanation, thanked me emotionally, and shook my hand. As he did, he tried to slip me a ten-dollar bill.

That was too much. I handed back the money and told him I had enjoyed caring for his wife and really didn't feel right taking his money. Pedro looked hurt, but then said quickly, "Do you ride a bike?"

That took me back a little. I admitted that I occasionally did.

"Good," said Pedro. "I'm the manager of a bike store down on Twelfth Street. I want to give you a bike, a nice ten-speed racer. My boss'll give me the bike free, so it won't cost me anything."

If I looked as I felt, I looked highly dubious.

"If you don't let me," said Pedro firmly, drawing himself up to his full height, "I will be very insulted."

I gave up and said I'd accept the gift, and thanked him.

"Oh, don't thank me," said Pedro. "It's the least I can do, after you saved my son's life."

I sighed. Right behind both temples, my head began to pound.

There must be thousands of women who are as convinced as Lucy was that prompt action by their obstetricians saved their babies' lives after the heartbeat had "stopped." As a conservative estimate, I'd guess that 99 percent of them are as wrong as she was. On the other hand, there have to be many more thousands of women who never took their babies home because the heartbeat really did stop, and it was not detected soon enough. Today many fewer of these errors occur, thanks to the development of sophisticated electronic monitors which provide a continous recording of heartbeat via electrodes applied to the fetal scalp. The very earliest irregularity of the heartbeat becomes immediately obvious and, where necessary, delivery by forceps extraction or caesarean section can be carried out before excessive deterioration of the fetal condition has occurred.

With all the caesareans now being performed, a readily accessible operating room is a necessity. Consequently, most modern labor and delivery suites have their own operating rooms as an integral part of the unit.

This was not the case, however, at The Vue in 1965. The only operating rooms in the hospital were located up in a different tower from the one containing the labor suite. Therefore, to get from one place to the other, we had to take an elevator down to the main floor, go through the corridors to the base of the second tower, and then take another elevator up. On the face of it, this doesn't sound like an overwhelming burden, but elevator service being what it wasn't, the trip often took fifteen or twenty minutes. One day I timed it at thirty-three. On that occasion, the elevator down from the labor suite passed our floor six times before the operator condescended to stop for us.

The inevitable delay was annoying, but usually not significant. In doing most caesarean sections, a half hour one way or the other didn't matter. But this was not invariably true. Sometimes there were indications that the baby was in trouble and should be delivered immediately. In other cases delay would have hazarded the life of the mother, for example when unstoppable uterine hemorrhage was taking place.

Thus, once again thrown upon his ingenuity, the Bellevue house officer was forced to solve yet another problem in makeshift, but semiworkable fashion. We had learned that a doorway in the operating suite led directly out onto the roof. The next crucial bit of data was the fact that a similar portal opened to the roof from the top floor of the tower containing the labor suite. We added up two and two and arrived at the conclusion that we could cut out one of the elevator trips. All that was necessary was to run the patient on her stretcher across the open rooftop of Bellevue Hospital.

About ten o'clock of an April morning, a woman whose name I never did get the chance to learn was admitted in labor. As I prepared to examine her, her bag of waters ruptured with a bang sufficient to spray amniotic fluid all over the opposite wall.

I put on a glove and examined the patient, and to my horror discovered that the worst had happened. With the rupture of the amniotic sac, the umbilical cord had prolapsed from the uterus into the vagina. I could easily feel three or four loops of it there.

I counted the pulsations in the cord at 130 beats per minute, a normal rate. But the danger existed that the baby's head might descend into the pelvis, compress the cord, and cut off the baby's supply of blood and oxygen from the placenta. Therefore I briefly explained the situation to the patient, apologized in advance, and extended my intravaginal hand tonsilward, to keep the baby's head high and off the cord. Then, at the top of my lungs, I bellowed out the two words that produce a frenzy in every delivery room in Christendom:

"PROLAPSED CORD!"

Nurses, doctors, and aides materialized as if by spontaneous generation. No one said a word; the routine was down pat. One nurse hastily shaved the patient's abdomen. A resident scanned the prenatal record for any information that might be worrisome in regard to the upcoming section. Another resident passed a tube into the patient's stomach to suck out the food and gastric juice that might otherwise enter the lungs during administration of anesthesia. Someone else called to alert the operating room. And through it all, I stood with my hand holding up the fetal head.

The chief resident strode into the room and took in the frantic scene. "What's the heart rate?" he said brusquely.

"I'm getting 130 a minute and steady," I said.

"Good," he said. "Let's go."

The shaving nurse swiped at a few stray strands of pubic hair.

"Come on," the chief barked. "I said, let's move it."

A hideous thought began to dawn on me. "How am I going to keep the head up, running alongside the stretcher?" I asked.

"You can't," the chief answered. "It's impossible. Get up on the stretcher and lie down."

I looked first at the patient and then back at the chief. "There's no . . . room next to her on the stretcher," I faltered.

"Then I guess you'll have to get on top of her," said the chief.

I stood frozen in place. Was he pulling my leg?

"Come on, God damn it, get up there," roared the chief. "Or do you want to wait till the cord stops pulsating?" His tone was harsh, but there was a little smile around the corners of his mouth. Who says fraternity initiations are dead?

I climbed aboard my incredulous patient, set my hand and arm firmly in position, and the nurse covered the two of us with a sheet. Then the chief and the senior resident wheeled the stretcher out of the labor suite and into the corridor. At every turn, I swayed and rocked perilously, but falling off was not my central worry. I just prayed I wouldn't see anyone I knew.

The senior resident pushed the emergency buzzer on the elevator, and not more than four minutes later the doors opened and we were being whisked to the top of the tower. My rigidly held forearm was beginning to throb in syncopation with the beating of the cord.

We flew off the elevator and began our journey across the roof. We shot around a corner, the sheet blew off, and I threw my free hand around the patient's neck or I'd have been a goner. That's when it happened. There was a gang of workmen scraping paint off the wall, and as we went past, they dropped their scrapers and stared at us in a unit. A cigar fell out of one gaping mouth.

A breathless "Jesus Fuckin' Christ!" floated after us as we zoomed through the doorway and into the operating area. The senior resident snickered and the chief guffawed. I didn't even smile, if for no reason other than I was in agony. Spasms of pain were shooting up from my wrist to my armpit.

As they shifted the patient to the operating table, I was able to get off her and stand up, but I still had to keep my hand in place, lest the head descend. If truth be known, by that time, I no longer cared whether the head descended, stayed in place, or even flew around in concentric circles. I even felt a little sorry I had started the whole thing. I was afraid my whole arm was going to fall off, and afraid that it might not. Compared to my assignment, that little Dutch boy at the dike had a picnic.

But I stayed in place until the other residents cut the woman open and extracted the screaming baby. At that point I fled out of the operating room even faster than I had come in. Frantically massaging my tingling arm, I headed down the hallway toward the elevator. No power on earth could have gotten me to walk back across the roof, past that platoon of goggling paint-scrapers. I cringed as I thought how I must have looked, lying on top of that woman, with my hand up to the elbow in—my God, I couldn't stand it! It was weeks before I could again examine a woman who had ruptured her bag of waters without feeling utter panic.

During the past one hundred years, there have been two truly major advances in obstetrical practice. Caesarean section has been one; the other, oxytocin.

Like caesarean section, oxytocin constitutes a means of expediting delivery. It is a hormone, normally secreted by the pituitary gland, and it can be synthesized. When administered to a woman in labor, it makes the uterus contract with greater force.

A hundred years ago, when uterine activity was weak and labor ineffectual, that meant real trouble. There were no good therapeutic options. The options then in vogue for stimulating uteri were either useless or did their job too well, producing such vigorous contractions that the baby would die and the uterus often would rupture. Caesarean section meant almost certain death for the mother. Consequently, labor often dragged on for three or four days, or even longer. Finally, with the mother exhausted, dehydrated, and infected, her attendant would have no choice but to reach in and pull the child out of the woman by brute force, a procedure which too often served as the *coup de grace* for both principals.

By the mid-1950's, however, the physiology and chemistry of oxytocin had become well understood, and it was then possible to do something about a lazy uterus. A small quantity of oxytocin could be mixed into a bottle of sugar water and administered intravenously. The faster the infusion rate, the more vigorously would the uterus contract. Hence a flow rate could be established that would produce a physiologic level of uterine activity to overcome a desultory labor.

In 1961, the Bellevue attitude toward oxytocin was one of caution. The dangers of the earlier uterine stimulants had not been forgotten; in addition, some of the oxytocin pioneers had used the drug indiscriminately, with unfortunate results. So we used oxytocin when we had to—but we knew that we'd damn well better be able to prove we *really* had had to.

On my very first day as a third-year medical student on obstetrics, I was assigned to help care for a seventeen-year-old who had come to the hospital almost with her first contraction. I sat at the bedside, compulsively timing the pains for hours on end, but nothing very much happened in the way of getting the baby delivered. The resident came in and broke her bag of waters, hoping that this act of aggression might stimulate and accelerate her labor, but she merely continued along her non-progressive way.

After eight hours of this, I began to feel punchy. By twelve hours, I was frankly hostile, and by sixteen hours, I was a raging misogynist. At eighteen hours, the first-year and senior residents came in and shook their heads sagely. My heart leaped: Might they be about to section her?

Not a chance. Down we went for X-ray pelvimetry, which demonstrated that the girl's pelvis was more than adequate for delivery of a normal child. The two residents studied the films at great length.

"What do you think?" asked the first-year resident. "Time for a little oxytocin?"

"I suppose," answered the senior. "But we'll have to check it out with the chief."

An endless half hour later, the chief resident was on the floor, looking at the X-rays. "All right," he finally said. "You want to give her some oxytocin, huh?"

The two younger residents nodded.

The chief laughed. "You know we can't do it without the approval of the attending. And you know who the attending is today, don't you?"

The first-year resident looked dismayed. "Aw shit," he muttered. "Not Haskins?"

Now the chief resident nodded, still laughing.

Forty-five minutes later, the three residents led Dr. Haskins into the labor room. Haskins was an ancient-looking man with stooped shoulders, thin white hair, a tremendous gray mustache, and a pair of watery blue eyes behind horn-rimmed spectacles. He wore a bemused little smile.

Dr. Haskins shuffled over to the bed and laid a trembling hand on the patient's abdomen. After he had timed and calibrated a few contractions, he haltingly performed a pelvic evaluation. Then he turned to face the residents.

"So you think she needs oxytocin, do you?" he asked.

"We'd like to give it a try," said the chief.

"Well, let me tell you," said Dr. Haskins firmly. "Oxytocin can be a dangerous drug. A very dangerous drug. Why, all she needs is a little tincture of time. You know what I do in cases like this? Why, I just go out into the hallway and I smoke a big black cigar. And by the time I'm done, the patient is usually ready to deliver."

The first-year resident rolled his eyes at me. Then they all walked out, admonishing me to keep a good eye on her.

Dr. Haskins could have smoked every big black cigar between New York and Cuba and that girl still wouldn't have been ready to deliver. My eyelids kept fluttering shut, and my mouth came to taste like Saturday at the county dump. Night passed into morning, and my charge had been hard at it for thirty hours.

At that point the senior resident came into the room with a syringe in his hand. He took down a bottle of 5 percent dextrose in water, injected the contents of the syringe, and swirled the bottle around. Then he connected the bottle to the woman's intravenous tubing and started the mixture dripping slowly into her vein. He winked at me.

"Now you're gonna see some action, kid," he said.

"Oxytocin?" I asked.

"Uh-huh."

"I thought Dr. Haskins wouldn't let you use it," I said.

"That was last night," said the senior resident. "Today our attending is Bill Crawford. He's a younger guy, and he doesn't shit at the mention of the stuff. We just called him up and presented the case, and he gave us the okay over the phone."

While the resident was talking, the patient had a contraction. This was nothing less than miraculous. For thirty hours the contractions had been as weak as they could have been, but this one was a winner. The uterus became rock-hard, stayed that way for almost a minute, and then eased up. The girl, who up till then had been emitting a series of soft Ay's with each contraction, now let go a fell-blooded roar.

"Great," said the resident. "Now we're in business. You see how fast the oxytocin is dripping—eight drops a minute? Well, it's your job to keep it going at that rate. Not seven, and not nine. And make sure she keeps having good contractions, too." With that, he charged out of the room.

In no time at all I learned why he had run away so fast. In those days, intravenous drip-flow rates were notoriously variable, being altered with every minor movement of the patient's limbs. The order to maintain a steady flow was a water torture far more devastating than the famous Chinese one. Every five minutes or so, I had to line my watch up behind the drip chamber, count the drops, and note the number of elapsed seconds. Then, when it was going too fast or too slowly, I adjusted the flow meter. Invariably I'd overshoot the mark and be forced to readjust. By the time I was finished re-re-readjusting the flow rate, it would be time to count the drops again.

I came to hate that innocent patient with an unmentionable ferocity. I fervently wished I could shackle her arm from neck to fingertips so that she'd be unable to wiggle her extremity and screw up the flow rate. I rained curses down upon that nine-months-old moment of passion that was causing me so much misery. I despaired of ever being free of the woman.

But it was now a whole new ball game. The oxytocin drip was producing a series of brobdingnagian uterine contractions, the patient was yodeling, the cervix was dilating, and the baby was descending. Within six hours she was safely delivered. Although the baby was not born in the best of condition, he was resuscitated with relative ease.

In truth, at the end of the thirty-six-hour ordeal, none of the three of us—baby, mother, and obstetrician—was in very good shape. Today that wouldn't happen. The oxytocin would be given much earlier, and it's very doubtful that the labor would last as long as twenty-four hours. Even better, there now exist constant-flow infusion pumps to provide a continual, steady intake of oxytocin. The days of the watch and the drip chamber are no more.

Thus, in retrospect, the modern obstetrics of the early 1960's at The Vue doesn't look so very bright and shiny and up-to-date. Matter of fact, the present-day crop of residents absolutely shudders at the mention of some of the things we did. Imagine practicing obstetrics without a fetal heart-rate monitor or a constant-flow oxytocin pump, and with the operating room half a hospital away. They all consider themselves very lucky indeed to have been born late enough to be able to work under truly modern conditions.

Epilogue

It's been eighteen years since I first set eyes on The Vue, and twelve years since I left. During those twelve years I've taught and practiced medicine at five other institutions in five different cities, and at the moment I'm living more than three thousand miles from New York. Nevertheless, a part of my mind still seems to be at Bellevue.

More of my dreams are on location at The Vue than at any other single place. Furthermore, when my phone rings at night and I struggle upward through the mists, I sometimes think that it's a nurse calling from B-3 to tell me the messenger just wheeled in another L.O.J.L. with congestive heart failure.

I experience similar occurrences even during my waking hours. I may be walking along a hospital corridor in Seattle and suddenly find myself hurrying toward B-2 to answer a stat page. Then the flyspecked walls vanish just as abruptly as they had appeared and I continue in the direction of my real destination.

I also have patient-related *deja vu* experiences. When I see a patient with a particular disease, I frequently recall the individual at The Vue in whom I first encountered the condition. And not only the individual, but usually also her specific location on the ward, the outcome of her case, and the month of the year I treated her.

When I tell my Bellevue stories to non-medical people, I understand why they sometimes ask me, "Come on—did that *really* happen?" The reality of The Vue is a long way indeed from what they've seen on *Marcus Welby* and *Medical Center*.

"Yes," I assure them, "it really did happen. Every bit of it. That's the way it was at The Vue."

At that point, they are likely to ask me another question. "If it was all such a charge," they say, "why have you never gone back? Why didn't you finish your training at Bellevue and then stay there as an attending?"

Actually, there are a couple of answers to that. For one thing, I've had all I can handle of the quality of life, New York style. I think in order to spend a lifetime in that place, you have to be more than a little masochistic. For another thing, I believe it's unwise to remain to teach at the institution where you had your training. It takes much too long for your associates to admit that you're no longer wearing short pants.

So, I can't go back to The Vue again. But I sure am glad I once was there.

CPSIA information can be obtained
at www.ICGtesting.com
Printed in the USA
BVHW03s1214050918
526585BV00004B/153/P